Ultra Keto Burn

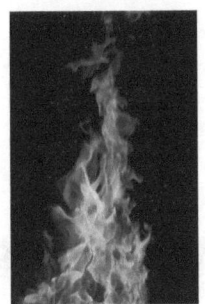

2 MANUSCRIPTS:

LOSE WEIGHT KETO AND KETO MINDSET

By Gabriel Walker

First Book

Lose Weight Keto

Easy guide to starting the Ketogenic Diet: Using Guaranteed Strategies and Methods to Help You Lose Weight, Burn Fat, and Rapidly Improve Your Mental Health

By Gabriel Walker

Lose Weight Keto

Easy guide to starting the Ketogenic Diet:
Using Guaranteed Strategies and Methods to Help You Lose Weight,
Burn Fat, and Rapidly Improve Your Mental Health

Table of Contents

Introduction

With the tremendous benefits that come with adopting a keto diet, many people are turning into it. But adopting a keto diet lifestyle only makes sense and becomes easy when you know what to do. Hence, it is not enough to decide to follow the keto diet; you need to be guided appropriately to make sure you are on the right part.

The desire to adopt a keto diet is not surprising as keto comes with tremendous health benefits. From losing weight to curing a range of disease like epilepsy and heart disease, the keto diet has proven very helpful. Overall, it helps maintain a healthy lifestyle free of excess weight and health challenges of excess weight. Over the years, many people have come up with different kind of meal plans to lose weight. Of all these plans, the keto diet has proven very effective.

This is why this manual is here as a guide. It will hold you by the hand in helping you start your journey into ketosis. We have meal plans that you can try as you go on. All in all, this manual will also shed light on what is ketosis and direct you on how to get there. Bear in mind, the ultimate goal of everyone adopting the keto diet lifestyle is to get to ketosis.

We urge you to remain faithful with the recommended ketogenic meal plans approved in this book. For it is when you are committed to the suggested meal plans that you can enter ketosis and reap the reward. All in all, get ready for a life changing experience that you will experience from adopting the keto lifestyle.

The keto diet involves adopting a meal low in carb, high in fat and with moderate protein. This could be pretty challenging for a couple of people. This is because there are challenges that will manifest as various signs when the body is transitioning into ketosis. Be rest assured this book is your ticket to ease the transition and reduce the effects.

Get ready for a complete overhaul in your health as I take you through this life-changing process.

Welcome

Chapter 1: Understanding Ketosis

Over the years, the spotlight has turned on the keto diet. This is not surprising as it is a meal plan that comes with abundant health benefits. The keto diet, a high fat and low carb meal plan, can turn your body into a fat burning machine. The surge in popularity of this meal plan can be attributed to celebrities and Hollywood stars that use it to stay in shape. The keto diet comes with many benefits from increased fat burning, to slowing down weight gain, to controlling blood sugar and reducing blood pressure.

Bear in mind that a keto diet is not a new found concept. It has been around as far back as 1920, almost a century ago when it was used to treat epilepsy. Then, researchers discovered that with elevated ketone levels in the blood, there were reduced epileptic seizures in sufferers (John M, 2013). With this, the keto diet was adapted as a treatment plan for kids and adults who do not respond to epileptic medications.

Ketogenic was coined form the 'ketones,' which led to keto, the shortened form. These are small fuel molecules that serve as a substitute for sugar in the body during a shortage of blood glucose. The production of ketones begins when humans feast on reduced levels of carb. Ketones also come from fat and serve as a powerhouse for the entire body, the brain especially. The brain which serves as the coordinating center of the whole body uses a lot of energy which comes either from the glucose or ketones.

Ketones in the body are produced in the liver from fats. These serve as a source of fuel for the entire body, the brain, especially.

The production of ketones in the body is called ketosis, a state of metabolism that should be desired by many people who wants to lose weight. The fastest way to get the body to ketosis is by fasting; however, fasting (staying away from food completely) could be pretty uncomfortable. With a keto diet, however, one can get to ketosis and reap the many health benefits of fasting even without fasting.

Switching to a keto diet means that the body is not powered by glucose, but fat. Unlike many other low carb diets, keto diets revolved around these macronutrients which are the source of 90% of the body calories. A drop in the level of body insulin spikes up the level of fat burned in your body. This is because fats are readily available; hence, they become the source of energy. With this, you will hardly go hungry since you get enough energy to stay focused all day

When the body is low in carb, the body transition to a metabolic state known as ketosis. This is when the level of ketones in the body rises, and the body breaks down glucose.

To shed weight, it is essential to burn fat. Besides that, getting the body to a state of ketosis does not come easy. Hence, you need to make it happen consciously. This is why your level of carb consumption in a day should drastically reduce. Some foods come with very high levels of carbohydrate like a banana (27grams of carb); hence take note of these foods and others in its category, it is also important to point out that one does not get to ketosis overnight. You will need a couple of days, days of dedication to the keto diet before getting to ketosis.

All in all, the keto diet is a low-carb diet which allows people to burn fat quickly since you concentrate more on eating fats, rather than carbohydrates. With the keto diet, your meal should contain a dietary plan of

- Fat in 60 to 70%
- Protein in 15 to 30% and
- Carbs about 5 to 10%

Types of Ketogenic Diet

Bear in mind that there are various types of the keto diet. However, they all revolve around reduced consumption of carbs and increased consumptions of fatty foods. A few of the types of keto diets are:

Standard keto Diet: this is the most common type of keto diet in which you eat a meager amount of carbs, (less than 50grams) per day. The ideal proportion is 75% fats, 20% protein, and 5% carbs.

Cyclical Keto Diet: If you want to commit to a cyclical keto diet, you will follow the standard keto diet meal indicated above 5 to 6 days a week. The carb intake during these 6 days is usually less than 50 grams. On the seventh day, you can eat as much as 150 grams of carbs – called the carb refeed day. The idea behind this is to cut back on the side effect that comes with restricting carb for a long time.

Targeted Keto Diet: While you also go with the standard keto diet, there is a slight difference. The difference is that 30 minutes before a high-intensity workout, you take extra carbs. The reason for this is apparent – for optimum performance

Dirty Keto Diet: With dirty keto, you will follow the recommended ratio of fats, carbs, and protein as suggested in the standard keto diet. The difference, however, is that you are at liberty to determine where your macros come from.

People Who Should Avoid the Keto Diet

Despite the effectiveness of a keto diet in bringing tremendous improvement to one's health, there are some group of people who should avoid the diet

People with Type 1 Diabetes: Type 1 diabetes patients are dependent on insulin. A keto diet could get their blood sugar level to dangerously low levels, which is terrible.

People with Eating Disorders: When you concentrate on a meal plan that eliminates a particular food group, there is a possibility of relapse in people with a history of eating disorder. Although Keto has proven pretty effective in helping to treat binge eating disorder, experts do not recommend this (Moira L, 2018). To treat binge eating disorder, you need a moderate, adequate, and regular intake of food without unnecessary ration.

People without Gallbladder: If your gallbladder has been removed, going on a high -ad diet will not help. This is because the gallbladder houses the bile, the body part that helps with digesting fat

People with Multiple Sclerosis: There are indications that a keto diet might not be safe in the long run for people battling with multiple sclerosis. There could also be side effects like constipation and fatigue.

All in all, bear in mind that a keto diet will not cure all disease. Also, going for the keto diet does not give the license to concentrate on all kinds of fats – there are unhealthy fats. Be sure to stay safe while on the diet

The next chapter will shed light on why you should consider the keto diet and the tremendous health benefits that come with this diet.

Chapter 2: Benefits of the Ketogenic Diet

Many people do attempt the keto diet for the sole purpose of losing weight. However, the keto diet comes with many health benefits. Keto diet gained wide acceptance and recognition because of its effectiveness in bringing about remarkable health changes.

By adopting the keto diet, some remarkable changes happen in the body that conditions it for tremendous health benefit.

A couple of the reasons you should try the keto diet are:

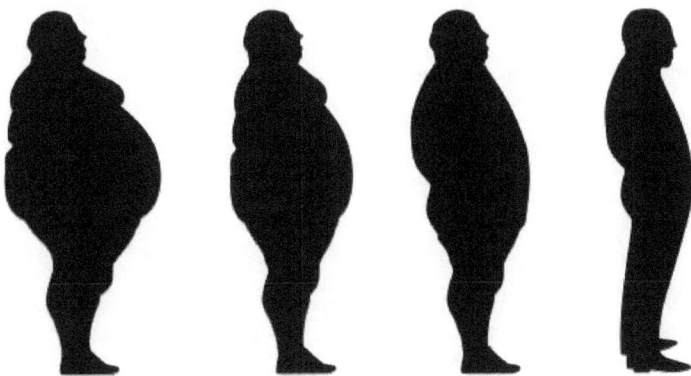

Weight loss

This is the number one reason why many people adopt the keto diet. At the onset of the diet, the body loses weight because of loss of water that comes from reduced carb intake. Hence, the body turns on fats stored in the liver since the consumption of carb has been limited.

Reduction in carb intake also reduces the level of body sugar. This translates to steady energy levels in the body. Besides, once people get used to the keto diet, they have a constant energy level such that they do not need to snack every couple of hours. Users are fuller with a lower level of hunger hence, reduced desire to eat.

Since your meal intake has changed, the body now burns fat for energy since glucose is scarce in the body.

This is how it happens:

On getting to ketosis, the levels of blood sugar and insulin drops. With this, the fat cells in the body let go of the water they have been holding on to. This is why a lot of people notice a significant weight loss on starting with the keto diet.

After this, the fat cells are in a better position to get into the bloodstream where they can find their way into the liver. In here, they get converted to ketones. This process goes on as long as you are on the keto diet.

Better Control of Your Appetite

This is one of the benefits of reduced carb intake. Your rate of hunger drastically reduces, and you do not suffer cravings like before.

Many people trying the keto diet discover that intermittent fasting becomes very easy. This is possible since hunger doesn't strike as it does before. Hence, you can go about your daily activities without rumbling from your stomach that you have got to eat

Improved mental Focus

Quite a lot of people have reported better memory and improved focus after getting on the keto diet.

When you concentrate on healthy fats, alongside omega-3 commonly found in seafood like tuna, salmon, and mackerel, you get to have a better mood with high learning capacity. This is not surprising as a fair percentage of the brain (15 to 30%) is made up of DHA, a fatty acid that gets increased due to the presence of omega-3 fatty acids.

Besides, getting into ketosis helps produce beta-hydroxybutyrate, a type of ketone. This is known to support and improve memory function.

Besides, one of the main issues with carbs as a source of energy is that it causes a rise and fall in the blood sugar levels. Due to the inconsistency of the source of energy, it becomes tasking for the brain to focus for long.

Getting into ketosis, however, makes the body turn on ketone for food. The source is consistent. Hence, you can focus for long.

Insulin Sensitivity

Excessively high levels of body insulin results in insulin resistance in the body. This can be addressed by using a keto diet. When you take meals high in carb, you are making the body's level of resistance to insulin to rise.

A keto diet, on the other hand, turns down the level of insulin in the body. This is understandable as you are now taking more of fat, a macronutrient that requires less insulin.

With a reduced level of insulin, your body can burn fat because excess insulin level works against the breakdown of fat. Hence, even a few hours drop in insulin level in the body encourages the breakdown of fat.

Control of High Blood Pressure

The number of people dealing with high blood pressure increases by the day. The problem is not really with increased blood pressure; the issue is that high blood pressure sets the stage for other horrible health condition like stroke, kidney failure, and heart disease.

There are, however, studies that buttress the fact that with a keto diet, you can get high blood pressure down, especially in people with type 2 diabetes or overweight people. (William S, 2015)

Cholesterol levels

With the keto diet, user can experience an improvement in the levels of cholesterol. What happens is that LDL levels decrease while HDL levels rise – which is expected and healthy

To know if you have a healthy cholesterol level, the ratio of total cholesterol to HDL matters. You can get this value by dividing the amount of your entire body cholesterol by your HDL level.

Your cholesterol level is healthy if you have a value of 3.5 and below. There is research that supports the fact that you can improve your cholesterol level with the keto diet.

Increased Energy level

The body cannot store much glycogen. As a result of this, you need to continually keep the level up to maintain a reasonable energy level.

In ketosis, however, this is not necessary as the body already has more than enough fat to work with. Hence, when you get to ketosis, hardly will the body run out of fuel. This translate to an optimum energy source

How beautiful it is if you do not have the urge to sink into your bed to relax after lunch!

This is the keto lifestyle!

Potential Health Risk of the Keto Diet

As impressive as the keto diet is, it doesn't come on a platter of gold. There are a few potential downsides that intending dieters need to know. The main one is that the diet is pretty challenging to stick with. According to a study in the Journal of Clinical Neurology, researchers sought for the rate of compliance among people on the keto diet and got 45%. According to Nisevich Bede

"The diet is pretty hard to follow because it's a complete shift from what you're used to,"

This can be attributed to the fact that your carb intake is significantly reduced. This makes you really, really hungry. Although the hunger subsides after a couple of weeks into the fast

Users should also bear in mind that there could be the possibility of flu-like symptoms. These manifest as fatigues, headaches, etc. This is commonly known as keto flu. Since you shed a lot of water weight on starting the keto diet, there is the possibility of dehydration. This could make keto flu worse. This is why staying hydrated is very important.

Other common health risks are a deficiency in some minerals and vitamins, kidney stones, reduced density bone density, etc. The reason for this is because there will be nutritional deficiency when you eliminate some classes of food like legumes, fruits, and whole grains. When you are short on fiber, for instance, there is a high chance you experience constipation.

To get around these risk associated with the keto diet, we recommend planning your need very well. This is important to ensure that you are having an adequate intake of essential nutrients. This might be difficult to expect if you are not working with a registered dietician with vast knowledge in keto.

Some Mistakes to Avoid While on the Keto Diet

A ketogenic diet is a complete change of lifestyle. As a result, it could be a struggle for a couple of people attempting the diet. This is because there is an internal change going on in the body, alongside a change in lifestyle and eating habits.

Many people tried the keto diet and loved the effects, while other people, on the other hand, did not see any reasonable change. Lack of result might be attributed to a simple mistake while on a diet.

You might make a mistake if you are not properly guided, but the fact that you are reading this manual will guide you against such errors. Following the keto lifestyle is hard; hence, you want to make sure you are armed with the right information to make sure everything goes as expected.

With this in mind, we bring forth common mistakes that people are prone to while on the diet.

Using keto as a "Quick Fix"

One thing many people who want to adopt the keto diet need to understand is that it is a lifestyle. Hence, it will not work if you're going to use keto as a quick fix for your weight or other health issues.

This is not to say that there will not be changes or effect at all, but the changes will not be long term. Besides, if you have any substantial change, you cannot expect to switch back to your formal eating habits and expect the changes to last. Hence, falling right back to your old eating habits will translate you right back to square one.

There are various types of the keto diet. As explained in the previous chapter, you can attempt the cyclical keto if the standard keto proves too hard. Bear in mind you are committing to a lifestyle change, and you have to be ready to stick to it long term.

That is how it works

Staying Away from Fats

Over the years, we have been made to believe that fat is the 'bad guy.' However, the irony of the matter is that keto diet makes you eat fat to lose fat, yes it is an irony, but it works.

Many people might marvel at the number of fats they have to eat when they calculate their macros. This is expected as a transition into ketosis is only possible with a massive amount of fats. Ideally, you should eat around 75% fat. This is a high amount, we admit, but it is ideal for getting rid of stubborn body fats lurking around your body.

You should not be afraid of eating such amounts of fat. In the long run, you will see tremendous health benefits hence be sure to flow along with the basics of the diet.

Concentrating on the Wrong fats

Alongside the last point, you have got to be sure that you are eating the right fat. That you have to eat a large portion of fat is not a license to pop in all kinds of fats. Without a doubt, there are good fats, and there are bad fats.

Bad fats prevalent in today's society are processed foods; processed vegetable oils, etc. hence, be careful of these and avoid cooking with these oils.

On the other hand, we recommend saturated fats, polyunsaturated fats, monounsaturated fats, and trans fat -natural ones. These are the types of fats that will aid your journey into ketosis.

With these types of fats, you will be sure to get the necessary amount of fat requirements while staying away from bad fats.

Eating Excessive protein

Okay, you are staying away from carbs, and you thought to compensate it with the intake of protein. Yes, that is fine, but the issue with this is that you will not get what you want. With excess protein, the body will have a negative reaction during fasting.

The body needs a certain amount of protein while adopting the keto diet lifestyle. Excess protein will be converted to fats, which is not needed. Bear in mind that part of the reason for keto diet is to get rid of fat hence adding another food that converts into an excess layer of fat is not worth it.

To avoid this, just concentrate on your macros. Be sure to eat based on your macros, and there will not be any class of food in excess.

Not taking Enough Water

Adopting the keto diet will make your body lose a lot of water. This explains why you have to make it a priority to stay hydrated. However, many people do not really focus on this.

Keto diet makes you lose not only fluids but electrolytes which you can easily replenish via the intake of water. Water deficiency in the body will make the body store a lot of fat, which is against what you want to achieve.

Besides, you need to be updated to ensure that your body organs are in top condition, well equipped to go about their normal activities.

Even if you do not like drinking water throughout the day, you have to. With the keto diet lifestyle, we recommend a gallon of water intake per day. This does not need to be overwhelming, as small sips can quickly add up to this with time.

Not Adding Variety to Your Meals

Without a doubt, a keto diet already places some level of restriction on the classes of food you can take many people, due to this, restrict themselves to a certain set of food every time. However, this does not mean you cannot experiment with varieties of recipes, as long as it is keto friendly.

That is part of the reason you have this keto diet manual, to expose you to as many keto recipes as possible. It is understandable to like a few sets of food. However, for optimum result, you should mix things up. There are keto recipes which you will get to experiment with later in this manual. This will not make the keto lifestyle journey boring in any way.

Be sure to include low carb veggies and fruits as well. This is because all the recipes will not have vegetables.

Be sure to experiment with varieties. It could be worse to concentrate on the same set of food every time. The disadvantage is glaring, with time, you will get fed up

Obsessing With the Scale

We understand that the ultimate goal of many on the keto diet is to lose weight. Bear in mind that you did not pack all the pounds of fat in a day; hence, they will not leave in a single day. Besides, the weight loss process is a journey which will take its time.

Checking the weight every now and then is a recipe for disaster. This might get you discouraged when things do not move as planned. Significant weight loss happens over a days and weeks, not hours.

However, be rest assured that if you follow everything as laid down, the meal classes in the right proportion, keeping hydrated and following your macro intake, your weights will reduce gradually.

Hence, the best idea is to check your weight once a week, And if you cannot keep your excitements down, check it twice a week. This will help you see the progress you are making with this new lifestyle of yours.

These keto mistakes can surely be avoided. To be forewarned is to be forearmed. Be sure to keep them in mind as you plan for the new lifestyle ahead of you

Chapter 3: What is Ketosis and How to get to Ketosis

Over the years, the basics of many fad diets out there teach us to restrict calories, have more workouts, and reduce fat intake for us to lose weight. However, many people have realized that the result of this is hardly effective.

Since the rate of obesity is rising geometrically, especially in developed counties, there has been research into healthy ways to lose weight. One of such is the keto diet. As it has been established in previous chapters, the keto diet not only produces weight loss but other tremendous health benefits for people who follow it.

The keto diet instructs users to eat meals high in healthy fats, moderate protein, and a limited amount of carbs per day. The aim of this is to get users to a metabolic state called ketosis. Entering into ketosis is the highlight of the keto diet. This is because users will not get the health benefits of the diet without getting into ketosis.

What is Ketosis?

Ketosis is a state you get to as a result of following the keto diet. In the body, you get into ketosis when the level of glucose from carbs drastically reduces. This forces the body to switch to another source of fuel – fat. While many people dread fat because it has been associated with excess weight and heart disease, it is a good source of energy in the absence of carbs.

When glucose is not available to fuel the body cells, the body looks for another source of fuel. This is when it burns fat for the production of ketones. As soon as the levels of ketones in the blood get to a certain point, the body gets to ketosis. This fosters a quick and consistent weight loss until you achieve healthy body weight.

In summary, here is ketosis and how to achieve that:

- A drastic reduction in the availability of glucose in the body, and all its sources like fruits, grains, starchy veggies, etc.

- The body seeks for an alternative means to keep up with its function - fat. This comes from food like avocado, salmon, coconut oil, etc.

- Since the primal source of fuel is not available, the body burns fat, which triggers the production of ketones in the blood.

- When your blood ketone levels get to a specific state, the body gets to a metabolic state called ketosis

It is the liver that breaks up fats into glycerol and fatty acid through a process known as beta-oxidation. In the body, we have three main ketone bodies produced in the liver, which are water soluble. They are acetone, acetoacetate, and beta-hydroxybutyrate.

Furthermore, the body breaks down these fatty acids in substance that powers the body called ketones that travels through the blood. The body breaks down fatty acid via a process called ketogenesis. This triggers the release of acetoacetate, a particular ketone that supplies energy.

With this, your body is powered by ketones moving around the body. This changes your metabolism such that you can burn fat quickly. With the ketogenic diet, you get to remain in this fat burning state. Since you achieve this via a low carb diet, you can no longer eat foods like bread, cereals, grains, and other processed foods. You now concentrate on foods like starchy vegetables, fish and butter.

Many people wonder how long it takes to get into ketosis. This depends on a couple of factors, but mainly on how limited your carb intake in, alongside some other variables that are not in your control like medical history, genetics, body composition, and energy needs. However, in a couple of weeks, your body should get to ketosis if you follow the keto diet strictly.

Some Signs You are in Ketosis

It is easy for some people to ease into ketosis because they can adjust to the lifestyle in a couple of weeks, a month tops. This happens with a few negative symptoms associated with the early stage of ketosis. It is common for your body to react when entering into ketosis. This is because your metabolism is changing.

Popularly known as keto flu, it could be a challenge for people starting out on the keto diet at first. This triggers some side effect that could stay for a week or two. The bright side, however, is that this goes away with time. As soon as your body starts getting used to being in ketosis, the symptoms decreases.

A few of the things you will likely experience as your body transition to ketosis are:

- Excessive tiredness
- Difficulty sleeping
- Extreme cravings for sugar and carbs
- Digestive issues such as constipation and bloating
- Being irritable
- Headaches and migraines

- Bad breath

This is what the initial phase of getting into ketosis will look like. On the bright side, you will likely notice some health improvement with time. Your appetite will reduce, and many of the positive benefits of the keto diet we discussed in the previous chapter. Those are indications you have positively transition to ketosis.

Experts on keto diets have declared that nutritional ketosis is measured by the levels of ketones in the blood, which is usually between 0.5 to 3.0 mM. Some people have agreed that 1.5 – 3 mmol/L is "optimal ketosis," which will trigger weight loss. People differ in regards to the exact amount of macronutrient they need to keep them in the range specified while giving them the ability to feel at their best.

You can also measure the levels of ketones in the breath, urine, or blood to determine if you are in ketosis. There are many ways to do this:

Blood ketone Meter: With the use of test strips, you can get an accurate measure of the BHB ketones in the blood. They are pretty reliable, and you can get them online to help know if your macronutrient consumption is in the correct ratio.

Urine Strip Tests: there are cheap urine strips which you can use to measure ketone levels is simple to use and cost-effective

Breathalyzer: You do not need a piece to measure ketones through your breath. The result might, however, not be as accurate as of the other two above.

Simple Tips to get into ketosis fast

We have established that when the body gets into ketosis, the body turns on fat as its source of fuel rather than glucose. The breakdown of fat in the body fills the blood with ketones. These ketones exit the body via the urine.

Achieving a state of ketosis requires some effort. This is why this section will shed light on simple, ways to get your body into ketosis fast.

Increase Workout

You can enter ketosis by increasing your physical activities. This is because the more energy you use for your daily activities, the more food you will need to replenish it. With exercise, the levels of glycogen in the body gets depleted, which gets renewed on eating carbs.

With the keto diet, however, you will not be replenishing the glycogen store since your intake of carb is reduced. Bear in mind that it could take a little while for the body to get used to fat for energy rather than glycogen. This could express itself in the form of fatigue as the body adjusts.

Drastically Cut Down the Intake of carbs

Since the body does not get enough supply of carbs, it is forced to act on fat, instead of sugar, as its primary source of fuel.

Hence, in trying to get to ketosis, we recommend limiting carb consumption to at most 20 grams per day. This will foster weight loss, help keep your blood sugar level in check while keeping your heart in good condition.

Short term fasting Period

One of the easiest ways to get to ketosis is via fasting. Many people find out that between meals, they could get to ketosis. Intermittent fasting as well, a short term fast interval, might also induce ketosis

There are cases a doctor might recommend a long period of fasting. It is advisable to be in touch with your dietician before deciding on any prolonged hour of fast.

Kids with epilepsy are at times made to fast for at least 24 hours before they commence the keto diet. This helps ease the transition into ketosis and the reduction of seizures.

Increase Consumption of Healthy Fats

You can improve your ketone levels when you eat a lot of healthy fats. Most, if not all, ketogenic diets have 80% of their calories from fat. The type of keto diet employed in treating epilepsy has up to 90% of fat.

Bear in mind; however, excess fat intake does not translate to higher ketone levels. You also, need to concentrate on high-quality fats only since the majority of your meal is made of fat. We recommend fats from sources like oil butter, avocado oil, butter, lard, and tallow, etc.

If your goal of following the keto diet is to lose weight, be sure to reduce your overall calorie consumption.

Maintain Optimum Protein level

You need a certain level of protein as well, although in minimal quantities. The keto diet used to treat epilepsy patients has a very limited amount of carbs and protein to boost ketone levels. We, however, do not advise cutting back on protein because it is not a healthy practice.

You need enough protein to equip your liver with enough amino acid, which helps in the process of gluconeogenesis, meaning "forming new glucose."

This is the process in which the liver provides glucose for the organs and body cells that cannot use ketones for fuel, for instance, the red blood cells and part of the brain and kidney. Also, you need optimum protein level to keep the muscle mass intact since there is a drastic reduction in carb intake.

Bear in mind that losing weight will result in the loss of fat, alongside muscle. When you take adequate protein with your keto diet, you get to preserve your muscle mass.

To know your protein need while on the keto diet, do multiply your healthy body weight (in pounds) by 0.55 to 0.77 (which in kilogram is 1.2 to 1.7Kg). Hence, if your ideal body weight, for instance, is 100 pounds, you should aim for a protein intake of 55 to 77 grams per day.

Consume More Good Salt

There is a couple of misconception about salt. This has made a lot of people struggle with the right amount of salt intake. This can be attributed to the excess carb ration which pumps up our insulin level. The kidney holds on to sodium because of excess insulin, which leads to a high Sodium and potassium ratio.

The keto diet, low in carb, helps reduce our levels of insulin. As a result of this, the body gets to pass out more of sodium as waste. Through this, we can get low Sodium to Potassium ratio. You can increase your intake of salt via any of the following:

- Use enough pink salt in your meals

- Consume more of organic broth

- Use sea vegetables like nori and help in your dish

- Take cucumber and celery – they are rich in natural sodium and low in carb

Use MCT Oil

One of the essential ingredients to get you into ketosis fast is high-quality medium chain triglyceride (MCT) oil. This is because it encourages the consumption of protein, which will keep you in ketosis.

If your diet is full of long chain fatty acids, 85% of the calories will be from fat. With MCT oil, you can get this level down to 65%. This is because it is easier for the body to digest MCT into ketones and used as energy.

It should be pointed out that MCT oil is not the same as coconut oil. While MCT oil comes from coconut oil, it contains some compounds that make it stand out. You can cook with MCT oil and even add it to drinks

KETOSIS EXPLAINED

TRADITIONAL DIET	KETOSIS DIET
High Carb	**High Fat**

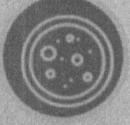 **GLUCOSE LEVELS RISE**

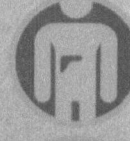 **GLUCOSE LEVELS FALL**

 **PANCREAS SECRETES INSULIN**

 **LIPASE RELEASES TRIGLYCERIDES**

INSULIN MOVES GLUCOSE INTO CELLS

FATTY ACIDS TRAVEL TO THE LIVER

ENERGY IS CREATED

LIVER PRODUCES KETONES INTO ENERGY

Do I have to spell this out for you? ☐

Chapter 4: Food to Eat and Foods to Avoid

There are many people without a clear direction on what to eat and what to stay away from while having the keto diet. This part of the book will shed more light on this. Being on a diet could be pretty hard, especially when you have no clue what you should eat and stay away from. We will give you an in-depth breakdown of the foods that can help you get to ketosis fast

Fats and Oil

When trying the keto diet, the bulk of your food will be fats; hence, it makes sense to start with it. In making your choice, keep in mind what you like and do not like. You can tweak fats in various ways to spice up your meals like sauces, dressings, etc.

The body needs fat to thrive, the right kind of fats. In a keto diet, we encourage some specific types of fats. There are various types of fats in different foods, but you can easily stay away from unhealthy fats.

Saturated Fats: Examples are ghee, butter, lard, and coconut oil. They are recommended.

Monounsaturated Fats: Samples are avocado, olive, and macadamia nut oils. They are also good.

Polyunsaturated Fats: We advise against processed polyunsaturated fats like margarine. However, you can take naturally occurring polyunsaturated fats found in animal protein and fatty fish.

Trans fat: these are processed fats that have been altered chemically. We advise you to stay away from these completely. All forms of hydrogenated fats like margarine should be avoided.

Monounsaturated and saturated fats like avocado, nuts, egg, butter, and coconut oil are stable chemically and do not trigger inflammation in many people. They are good.

There should be a balance between your omega 6's and omega 3's. Hence, focus on foods like tuna, salmon, shellfish, and trout. You can take a small fish oil supplement if you do not like fish. We also recommend krill oil as a substitute for omega 3.

Be careful about the amount of sea-based foods and nuts you take since their levels of omega 6 could be quite high. Foods in such categories are walnuts, sunflower oil, corn oil, almonds, etc. To keep your omega 's at the normal range: concentrate on fatty and animal fish, reduce snacking, and be wise with dessert items.

With essential fatty acids, the body gets the needed boost for its vital functions. The problem, however, is that when on a diet, they could be out of balance. Some fat and oil fit for a keto diet is

- Olive Oil

- Egg Yolks

- Avocados

- Avocado Oil

- Mayonnaise

- Cocoa Butter

- Coconut Oil

- Macadamia/Brazil Nuts

- Coconut Butter

- Butter/Ghee

Proteins

We recommend choosing a protein food source that is pasture and grass-fed. This is essential to limit intake of bacteria and steroid hormone. Below is a list of proteins that are fit and perfect for a keto diet. However, you should eat a regulated amount of protein.

As regards poultry, we recommend choosing dark meat if possible, because it contains much fat content, compared to white meat. Red meat does not have too much restriction. Be careful with sausages and cured meats as they could come with added sugars and processed ingredients.

In eating meat, you have to be careful of your protein intake. Excess protein in your diet could reduce the production of ketones in the body and an alternate increase in glucose production. The aim is nutritional ketosis. Hence, you need to be smart with protein.

Some proteins fit for the keto diet are:

- **Fish:** We recommend everything caught in the wild such as cod, catfish, mackerel, salmon, trout, flounder, halibut, tuna, salmon, and mahi-mahi. Be sure to concentrate on fatty fish.

- **Poultry:** Pheasant, duck, chicken, and quail.

- **Beef:** Steak, roast, stew meat, ground beef.

- **Pork**: ham, ground pork, tenderloin, pork loin, etc. be careful of added sugar and concentrate on fattier cuts.

- **Shellfish**: lobsters, oysters, mussels, squid, and crabs.

- **Offal/organs:** tongue, liver, heart, and kidney. Offal is an excellent source of nutrients.

- **Whole Eggs:** We recommend going for the ones from the local market. It could be prepared in many ways: poached scrambled fried and deviled.

- **Bacon and Sausage:** be sure to stay away from sugar or any extra filer additions by checking out the labels

- **Nut butter:** We recommend natural, unsweetened nuts, the fattier version if possible. This is macadamia nut butter and almond butter. Be smart with legumes as they are high in Omega 6.

For protein, always keep in mind that moderation is essential.

Vegetables and Fruits

We have as well made a list of fruits and vegetables fit for consumption while having the keto diet. It is important to note that some fruits and vegetables contain carbs in large quantity. Hence, it is essential to reduce the intake of such.

Vegetables are essential while on the keto diet. However, be careful about veggies as some come with high sugar content. Hence, you have got to be smart with your choice.

For a ketogenic diet, we recommend vegetables high in nutrient and low in carbs; in other words, the dark and leafy vegetables. Classes of spinach and kale also fit into this category.

We also recommend cruciferous vegetables grown above the ground, which are green and leafy. We recommend going for the organic type, though, due to the reduced level of pesticides. For vegetables that grow below the ground, be smart in consuming those. However, an idea of their carb level will be helpful.

All in all, there is no hard and fast rule when it comes to taking vegetables on the keto diet. You have got to be careful and mindful of the carb content. In adding any vegetables to your meal, be sure to **limit** these types:

- **Higher Carb vegetables**: Onions, parsnip, mushroom, and squash are in this category.

- **Berries:** This is blackberries, blueberries, and raspberries.

- **Nightshades:** peppers, tomatoes, and eggplants

- **Citrus:** lime, lemon and orange juice in water

- Completely Stay away from bananas, starchy vegetables, and large fruits like potatoes.

- All in all, it is a general fact that fruits and vegetables that grow underground come with a higher amount of fat. Hence, take them in a controlled and limited amount.

Dairy Products

There are dairy products that are fit for consumption while on the keto diet as well. However, the same rule applies, be mindful of the carb content since the idea is to have a reduced intake of carb in general, irrespective of the source.

Diary is an excellent addition to meals while on the keto diet. However, your levels of dairy must be moderate as you want to consume more proteins, vegetables with fats and oil.

We advise going with raw and organic dairy foods if you can get them. Dairy that has been processed does come with a magnified amount of carbs, which is not the best idea. Besides, we advise full-fat products over low fat or fat-free since the fat content will be high.

For lactose intolerant people, we recommend great aged dairy products since they have reduced lactose. Some dairy products fit to eat while having the keto diet are:

- Heavy whipping cream and Greek yogurt
- Hard Cheese such as cheddar, feta, Swiss, etc
- Soft cheese like blue, brie, Colby, mozzarella and Monterey Jack, etc.
- Spreadable like cheese, sour cream, crème Fraiche, cottage cheese, cream cheese, etc.
- Mayo alternative and Mayonnaise that has dairy

Dairy can be an additional source of fat while on the keto diet. With meals like sauces, fatty side dishes such as creamed spinach, etc. However, bear in mind that these classes of food lack in protein. Always remember this when eating them along with a protein meal.

A couple of people could have reduced weight loss while taking excess cheese. Hence, if you notice your weight loss has slowed, we recommend checking how much dairy you consume.

Nuts and Seeds

You can also consume a number of nuts and seeds on a keto diet, But as with other classes of food, be sure to be careful of the carb content. We recommend roasting nuts to get rid of any anti-nutrients. Stay away from peanuts since they are legumes and not recommended on the keto diet food.

With raw nuts, you can add flavorings to your meal. You might choose to consume them as a tasty snack. This is, however, not recommended if you are after weight loss. Your insulin levels will generally rise and slow down the rate of fat burning in the long run

You can get good fats from nut but be sure to remember that they come with carbs that can add up pretty quick. Besides, some nut also comes with protein.

- **Nuts can also be high in Omega 6 fatty acids**; hence, be mindful of the amount you are taking in. In general, go for nuts low in carbs. The following can guide you when it comes to choosing nuts for eating while on the keto diet:

- **Fatty low carb nuts:** You can eat brazil nuts, pecans, Macadamia nuts to supplement fats

- **Fatty, moderate carb nuts**: almonds, walnuts, peanuts, hazelnuts, and pine nuts will help supplement for flavor

- **Higher Carb nuts**: Stay away from cashews and pistachios because of their excessive carb content. With two handfuls of cashew, you get the whole carb you should eat in a day

Rather than regular flours, you can go for nuts and seeds. They are standard on the keto diet and very common with keto diet desserts and baked recipes. Nuts are commonly used in almond flours while seeds are conventional on flaxseed meals.

In baking recipes, you can employ multiple flours to get a good texture. You can also combine and try various baking methods to get reduced carb counts in your recipes. It is also vital to bear in mind that we have multiple types of flours that act differently. For instance, the body quickly absorbs coconut flours, which require more liquid.

Water and beverages

We present some common forms of beverages that are allowed and recommended while on the keto diet. However, you should limit the consumption of restricted beverages.

Bear in mind that being on the keto diet drains water from the body. You lose a lot of water weight at first, which could cause dehydration. This is common when starting out the menu. However, you need to be extra prepared if you are prone to bladder pain or urinary tract infections.

Usually, it is best to drink eight glasses of water. This is useful while on the keto diet, but you need more. Bear in mind that a large percentage of the human body is made up of water; hence, hydration is critical to survival and optimum function of the body organs.

You might want to go for keto coffee in the morning to boost your energy levels. While this is good, moderation is key as well. Be sure to go easy on the caffeine as well as it could stall your weight loss process. If you must take caffeine, we recommend not taking more than 2 cups a day.

It is important to note that keto flu occurs as a result of dehydration and insufficient electrolytes in the body. This explains why drinking enough water is not negotiable as well as replenishing your electrolytes.

A list of the most popular beverages while on the keto diet are:

- **Water:** this is your ideal liquid to curb hydration. We recommend still or sparkling water

- **Broth**: combined with vitamins and nutrients, it is an excellent way to replace your energy as it helps kick start your energy.

- **Coffee:** helps with focus and mental clarity. It can also help improve the weight loss effect of the keto diet

- **Tea**: gives the same results as coffee. However, we recommend black or green tea if you do not enjoy a drink

- **Almond/Coconut milk**: we recommend the unsweetened version to replace your diary beverage

- **Diet Soda:** We advise limiting this as it can lead to sugar spike and cravings.

As evident, the keto diet is not as restrictive as you might be tempted to believe. There is much food you can choose, and your dish is only as limited as your creativity. All in all, in whatever you want to choose, be sure to be careful of the level of carb. To a large extent, it determines if you will get to ketosis. On the other hand, we also have a whole list of foods that you should stay away from if you are on the keto diet. The next section discusses this.

Foods to Avoid on a Keto Diet

We describe the classes of foods that should not be eaten or found in your recipes when going on the keto diet.

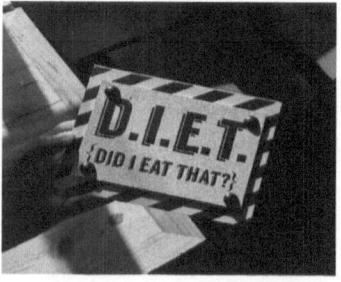

Starch and all its form

In abiding by a low carb diet, staying away from starch is critical. In our food today, the most significant source of carbohydrate is corn and wheat; hence, be on the watch out for them. However, in avoiding starch, you have got to be wary of all forms of flours (except nut flours) and grains. Starchy vegetables like beans and tubers are off the table as well.

Some forms of grains you should get off your food lists are:

- Corn
- Rice
- Sorghum
- Millet
- Rye
- Oats
- Quinoa
- Wild Rice
- Wheat
- Bran
- Bulgar
- Durum
- Wheat berries
- Amaranth
- Spelt
- White flour
- Triticale
- Arrowroot
- Semolina
- Flour
- Cornmeal

- Cottonseed

- Cassava

- Lentil

- Manioc

- Modified starch

If you have to bake, you can use low carb baking with ingredients like coconut flour, almond flour, etc.

All forms of Sugar

Even when not on the keto diet, sugar is not so healthy for the body. Besides, it wreaks untold havoc on the body that moderation is vital. Now when on a menu like a keto, it is important to limit sugar intake to very, very minute quantities.

Besides, you need to be smart about sugar as it comes in many names. Hardly will you see a product where the manufacturer will spell out sugar directly as part of the ingredients. It is masqueraded in various fancy names and comes in different forms as well. They give sugar many fancy names so that you will not suspect the amount of sugar that comes in a product. Hence, when buying your next packaged food, be on the watch out for the following:

- Brown sugar

- Barbados sugar

- Castor sugar

- Coconut palm sugar

- Date sugar

- Golden sugar

- Icing sugar

- Yellow sugar

- Raw sugar

- Grape sugar

- Brown rice syrup

- Carob syrup

- Corn syrup solids

- Sounds like syrup—

- Palm Sugar

- Golden syrup

- Diastatic malt

- HFCS

- Muscovado

- Panocha

- Corn syrup

- Caramel

- Scant

- Treacle

- Malt

- Florida Crystals

- Powdered sugar

- Invert sugar

- Corn Sugar

Be careful of sugars listed as their scientific names. Watch out for the following names, and it sounds like a chemical, scientific mumbo jumbo:

- Diatase

- Fructose

- Glucose

- Ethyl maltol

- Fructooligosaccharides

- Isoglucose

- Glucose solids

- Glucitol

- Lactose

- Galactose

- Maltose

- Levulose

- Dextrose

- Disaccharides

Do not be deceived, sugar is sugar, regardless of any fancy name that they give it.

Stay Away from bad fats

Fats are not created equal hence, on your next trip to the grocery store, be sure to review the set of ingredients on the packet. This simple act can help you stay away from artificial trans fats and processed vegetable oil.

As much as possible, stay away from trans fat that is produced artificially. You will likely see them as "partially hydrogenated" oil or vegetable in short. Also, all processed vegetables oil and margarine should be highly limited. The means of producing these oils are very unhealthy – commercially, they are dissolved in a solvent under high heat, deodorizers, and bleach. They come from a science experiment and not stable under heat. Stay away from them as much as possible. Be on the lookout for the following:

- Anything hydrogenated

- Anything partially hydrogenated

- interesterified oils

- Diglycerides

- Monoglycerides

- Margarine

- Processed vegetable oils

- Cottonseed

- Rice Bran

- Soybean

- Corn

- Canola

The sad part is that these classes of refined vegetable oils can be found in many products. Be sure to stay away from trans fat and check the ingredient list. Don't check the nutrition facts label. Some products might still have artificial trans fat in trace amounts which might not be reflected in nutrition fact labels. Because trace amount can quickly add up hence, double check a product.

Some foods like butter and meat also have trace amounts of naturally occurring trans fat, and this is not a cause for concern. It is the artificial one that is your enemy, and not the natural one.

Chapter 5: 10 Delicious Sample keto Recipes

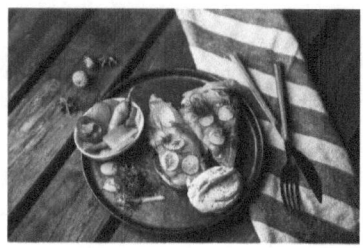

1. Coconut Keto Coffee

Ingredients

- Ghee – 1 tablespoon
- Coconut oil – half tablespoon
- Black coffee – 1 cup

How to prepare

Put all the ingredients in a blender and blend thoroughly

Serve appropriately

Recipe Notes

Servings: 1

Macros (per serving):

Calories: 179 kcal

Fat: 21 g

Protein, Net carbs, and Dietary fiber: 0 g

2. Keto Frittata

List of Ingredients

- Bacon – 4 slices

- Eggs – 6 large ones
- Baby Spinach – 4 ounces
- Shredded cheddar cheese – 1 cup
- Sliced mushroom – 1 cup
- Butter – 2 tablespoons
- Pepper – 2 tablespoons
- Salt – half teaspoon
- Heavy cream – a quarter of a cup

How to prepare

Preheat your over to 1800 C

Over the high heat, place a cast iron, preferably frying pan

Add your diced bacon and sauté into the frying pan.

Leave for about four minutes and add butter.

Get your sliced mushroom ready and pour in the pan

Sauté the entire mixture for about three minutes

Into the cooking mixture, add spinach and cook for two more minutes till it is wilted.

Remove from the heat and add some cheddar cheese into the pan

Get a mixing bowl, in it put cream, eggs, pepper, and salt

Whisk the entire mixture thoroughly till it is combines

Pour all the mixture into the pan and place in the over

Bake for 20 minutes

After this, it is ready for serving

Recipe Notes

Servings: 4

Macros (per serving):

Fat: 36 g

Protein: 21 g

Calories: 426 kcal

Total carbs: 3 g

Dietary fiber: Nil

3. *Lemon Black Pepper Tuna Salad*

List of Ingredients

- Dice one-third of a whole cucumber into small pieces
- Dice half of a small avocado into small pieces
- Lemon juice: 1 teaspoon
- Tune: 1 can
- Use salt and black pepper to taste
- Mustard: 1 tablespoon
- Mayonnaise: 1 tablespoon
- Salad green

How to prepare

With your cucumber already diced, mix it with lemon juice and avocado

Flake the tuna and mix with mayonnaise and mustard

Add the two mixtures together – tuna with cucumber and avocado

If you want, you can add salt to taste.

Serve and enjoy

Recipe Notes

Servings: 1

Macros (per serving):

Fat: 40 g

Protein: 45 g

Calories: 480 kcal

Total carbs: 11 g

Net carbs: 3 g

Dietary fiber: 8 g

4. White Lasagna Stuffed Peppers

List of ingredient

- Sweet pepper – 2 large, seeded and halved

- Garlic salt - 1 tablespoon

- Ground turkey – 12 ounces

- Mozzarella – 1 cup

- Ricotta Cheese – 1 cup

- Cherry tomato – 8 (optional though)

How to prepare

Raise your over to temperature as high as 205-degrees Centigrade

Put the halved sweet pepper into the baking dish and spread one quarter garlic salt in it

Unto the pepper, spread out the turkey. Sprinkle another quarter teaspoon of garlic salt.

Place the mixture in the oven and bake for about 30 minutes

Into the pepper, sprinkle the ricotta cheese and the mozzarella and the remaining garlic salt.

If you are using the tomato, slice it into the mixture

Bake for half an hour till the meat is well cooked, the pepper softens out, and the cheese becomes golden.

Serve into four plates and enjoy

Recipe Notes

Servings: 4

Macros (per serving):

Fat: 14 g

Calories: 281 kcal

Protein: 32 g

Net carbs: 6.5 g

Total carbs: 7 g

Dietary fiber: 0.5 g

5. Shrimp and Zoodles

List of Ingredients

- Butter – 1 tablespoon
- Shrimp – 1 pound
- Butter – 1 tablespoon
- Zucchini – 3 medium size
- Chopped garlic – 5 cloves
- Olive oil – 1 tablespoon
- Paprika - 1 teaspoon
- Lemon juice – 3 tablespoons
- Chopped parsley – a quarter cup
- Red Chili flakes – 1 pinch
- Pepper - ¼ tablespoon
- Salt - ½ teaspoon
- Use feta or parmesan for garnishing

How to prepare

You will need a zoodle device to make your zucchini. Spread it out on the double paper towels.

Spread a teaspoon of salt and roll up the towel.

Leave for a couple of minutes

Inside the pepper, add your shrimp, salt, paprika, and chili flakes

Get a large skillet, place over low heat

Add a tablespoon of butter and allow to melt.

Add a tablespoon of olive oil to the mixture

Add the shrimp and leave for about 3 minutes to cook and turn

Leave an extra 2 minute for the other side to cook

Remove from the skillet and put aside

Add garlic, red pepper, into the skillet and allow to cook for about 120 seconds.

Into the pan, add lemon juice and scrape it off the pan

Add the zoodles and sauté for an average of 4 minute

Into the skillet, add shrimp and some parsley

Stir while it is being cooked.

Serve into four plates

Recipe Notes

Servings: 4

Macros (per serving):

Calories: 210 kcal

Fat: 8 g

Protein: 25 g

Total carbs: 8 g

Net carbs: 6 g

Dietary fiber: 2 g

6. Keto Homemade ham

List of Ingredients

- Smoked boneless gammon – 2 pounds
- Chopped onions - 1 piece
- Chopped celery stalk – 1
- Garlic cloves – 1, bashed

- Black peppercorns – 2 teaspoons
- Whole cloves – 1 teaspoon
- Whole cinnamon stick – half
- Whole nutmeg – a quarter
- Salt – a quarter of a cup

How to prepare

Get a large pot, out the entire ingredients and add cold water

Boil the water and skim off the top foam with a spoon

Reduce the heat to the simmer, leave the pot cover ajar to facilitate slow evaporation

Simmer for 90 minutes

Leave for about an hour to allow the ham cool

Separate the liquid and place in a refrigerator.

It can be preserved for up to 7 days

Recipe Notes

Servings: 8

Macros (per serving):

Calories: 112 kcal

Protein: 20 g

Fat: 4 g

Net carbs and Dietary fiber: 0 g

7. Fresh Bell Pepper Basil Pizza

List of Ingredients for the Pizza base

- Mozzarella Cheese – 6 ounces
- Almond flour – half cup
- Psyllium husk powder – 2 tablespoon

- Egg – A large one

- Italian seasoning – 1 teaspoon

- Parmesan Cheese – 2 tablespoons

- Salt – half teaspoon

- Pepper – half teaspoon

List of Ingredients for the toppings

- Shredded cheddar cheeses – 4 ounces

- Tomato – a piece

- Marinara sauce – a quarter of a cup

- Bell pepper – two third

- Basil – 3 tablespoons

How to prepare

Preheat your oven to a temperature of 204 degrees Centigrade

Put the Mozzarella cheese in your microwave till it is melted

Put all the pizza base ingredients in the cheese and mix thoroughly

With a rolling pin, flatten the dough into a circle

Put the entire mixture in the oven for 10 minutes,

Get it out of the oven and spread the topping ingredient on top

Put it back in the oven and allow it to bake for an extra 10 minute

Recipe Notes

Servings: 4 (half pizza is 1 serving 2 pizzas of 4 servings.)

Macros (per serving):

Calories: 411 kcal

Fat: 31.3 g

Protein: 22.3 g

Net carbs: 6.5 g

8. Brownie Batter Mug Cake

List of Ingredients

- Almond flour – 1 tablespoon
- Flaxseed meal – 1 tablespoon
- Butter – 2 tablespoon
- A large egg
- Baking powder – half teaspoon
- Cocoa powder – 1 tablespoon
- Nut Zez Brownie Batter Almond Butter – one and a half tablespoon

How to prepare

Put the entire ingredient in a mug and mix

Microwave for about a minute

Leave it to cool and pour the content in a plate, leaving the mug upside down

To make the brownie flow out, tap the mug and enjoy

Recipe Notes

Servings: 2

Macros (per serving):

Calories: 242 kcal

Net carbs: 2.6 g

Fat: 23.3 g

Protein: 7.8 g

9. Low Carb Cheesecake Brownies

List of Ingredients for the brownie

- Salt – half teaspoon
- Almond flour – three quarter cup

- Erythritol – two-third of a cup
- Cocoa powder - two-third of a cup
- 2 large eggs

List of ingredients for the Cheesecake

- A large egg
- Vanilla extract – 1 teaspoon
- Erythritol – One-quarter of a cup
- Cream cheese – 8 ounces

How to prepare

Preheat the oven to 175-degree centigrade

With a parchment, line the bottom of an 8 by 8 pan

Spray cooking spray on the pan

Cream the sweetener and cream cheese together till it is smooth

Add the vanilla and egg and mix thoroughly till you achieve a cream and soft feeling

Melt the butter, add sweetener, salt, and cocoa.

Stir vigorously till the sweetener dissolves

As you stair, add the egg to the mixture one at a time

Add the almond flour slowly as you mix till it forms a good dough

Add two third of the brownie batter into your prepared pan

Dollop your cheese batter into the brownie

Pour the rest of the brownie batter.

Bake for like 23 minutes and keep an eye on it

Allow to cook and cut

Refrigerate it for about 10 minutes

It can be left in a refrigerator for 3 days

Recipe Notes

Servings: 16

Macros (per serving):

Calories: 155 kcal

Fat: 15 g

Protein: 4 g

Net carbs: 1.5 g

10. *Loaded Cauliflower Mashed Potatoes*

List of Ingredients

- Cauliflower – 1 head
- Garlic – 1 clove
- Butter – 3 tablespoon
- Salt – half teaspoon
- Pepper – one eight teaspoon
- Green onions
- Bacon – 4 slices
- Sour cream – 1 tablespoon

How to prepare

Heat a pot of water to boiling point and put the cauliflower in.

Reduce the heat and simmer for an average of 10 minute

Drain the water from the cauliflower

Get a food processor, add the garlic, pepper, salt, cauliflower, and sour cream

Process the entire mixture for about two minutes

Spread some cheese, green onions and crumbles on the top

It is best served warm

Recipe Notes

Servings: 4

Macros (per serving):

Fat: 22 g

Calories: 257 kcal

Protein: 7 g

Net carbs: 5 g

Chapter 6: How to Maintain the ketogenic Lifestyle

By now, you have all the tips needed for getting your body into ketosis. Bear in mind, and it is not enough to get to ketosis but to remain in ketosis as well. Hence, it is essential to arm yourself with crucial tips to help you maintain ketosis.

We discuss some of the essential tips below:

Concentrate only on keto Friendly Foods

The idea behind the keto diet is a meal very low in carb. However, the amount of low carb for the various individual is a factor of the daily carb limit. Hence, it is best to keep the net carbs below 25gram and total carb below 35 grams. This will enable you to reap the benefits of the keto diet.

Since your carb intake is limited, you have to be smart about food choices. Hence, you might have to ditch some of your favorite foods you have been used to over time. We do not even recommend all healthy fruits and vegetables. This is not to discourage you in any way, and there are other delicious recipes you will find interesting.

The previous chapters have done justice on the food that is recommended and not advised on the keto diet.

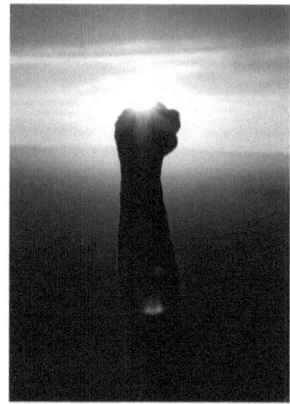

Track Your Macros

Many people hardly pay attention to the number of calories they eat. Besides, estimated calorie intake and actual calorie we eat is usually so different that we might be tempted to feel we are eating way less calorie.

We advise using a calorie tracking app and a scale to keep tabs on what you are eating. This method will help you know if you are consuming the right food amount as well as direct you on how to go about your weight loss.

You can get accurate info about the type of calorie you are taking by using a food scale. Many people base their calorie intake on guesswork, which can sometimes make you eat extensively. In buying a range, be sure to look for the following features

Presence of a conversion button: Most websites and calorie tracking apps use varieties of units. With a conversion button on your scale, you should be able to measure your food quickly. Most especially, we recommend going for a gram to an ounce or an ounce to a gram.

Tare Function: You should be able to have bowls, plates, and other utensils on your scale. This makes it easier to weigh things. There should be a tare function on it so you can place items on it

Removable Plate: There should be a removable plate to bring about easy cleaning. This is due to the possibility of having messy foods on your scale.

Tracking your food consumption the right way will help you focus on getting the result you want, keeping you in ketosis

Be careful of Your Environment

The type of food the world presents to us is way different from what our forefathers grew into. We are met with all kinds of foods that make it easier for the disease to attack and for people to pack excess weight. This was not what our forefathers had, which made it easier for them to have a long life and a lean body.

Processed foods are abundant in every corner, we watch it in commercials, and the smell attracts us. This triggers our brain to go for this tantalizing aroma, which comes so quickly. To make things worse, we eat way more than we need. This triggers weight gain. As a result of this, it is essential to do all in your capacity to make your environment keto friendly.

Some of the things we recommend are:

Keep only keto Friendly Food around: Hunger makes it so easy to cheat and feast on anything available. Hunger has a strong drive which acts irrationally and does not care about your weight loss goals. As a result of this, we advise you always to plan and make your home keto friendly. Let all carb-rich food be out of reach, and the healthy keto friendly food be within reach. Besides, keto food should want to go for should not require much preparation.

Always Plan Your meals Early: A plan makes it easy to stay on track and avoid temptation. There are keto friendly snacks and pre-made meals you can go for. All in all, your meal plan should give you the right amount of carb, fats, and protein in the recommended proportion

Avoid Easy foods that Might make You Binge: A convenient and tasty food is more natural to eat since it doesn't require much effort for preparation. Some people can go for an excess amount of a particular food, even keto food. As a result of this, we recommend not making an excessive amount of a food item at once. Hence, if it will be hard for you to control the urge to binge eat a particular food, restrict the amount you make such that making another will discourage

Concentrate only on Foods you can measure and track: Do not be tempted to include other instruments you will not be able to measure. It can get you off your macronutrient goals. A little extra oil and cheese here and there could shoot up your calorie to the point where it gets easy to gain weight.

Avoid Changing Your Plan Quickly

Your body will lose a ridiculous amount of water when you start keto, which manifests as weight loss. This will cause a change in the amount of calorie you need, and with time, there will be variation in the number of calories you need. With this, you will lose weight but not at a fixed pattern.

The implication of this is that some weeks will feel as if you are not losing weight. You might be discouraged by what the scale tells you. It is, however, important to stick with the plan as this helps long term weight loss.

You should aim for an average weight loss of 1 to 2 pounds per week. However, if you discover that you are not making encouraging progress, we recommend adjusting your lifestyle and diet choice. Take note of the following strategies

- Know your macro requirement and be sure it is deficient in calories. If you are after weight loss, make sure the deficit is high

- Make it a monthly strategy to calculate your macro needs monthly. Make this the plan you will stick with.

- Take breaks once a while from being in a calorie deficit, maybe once a week

- Track the food you eat and never cheat

- Attempt intermittent fasting

If the above strategy did not work, there might be a food allergy holding you back. Besides, it could also be that you are getting excess calorie from a hidden source.

Be Set for keto Flu and other keto Concerns

You have been so used to consuming carbs without restriction. Switching to a low carb food all of a sudden will be met with lots of revolt from your body. Many people will experience excess loss of minerals like sodium and water at first. Here are some of the keto flu you should prepare for dizziness, insomnia, confusion, stomachache, brain fog, irritability, nausea, and muscle soreness.

The best part is that by taking a lot of water, you will get rid of these symptoms. Hence, to be in ketosis for long, you have got to make it a habit to take lots of water

Use a Smart Meal plan

Following a meal plan is the best way to get and keep you in ketosis. This will reduce the overwhelming feeling from having to process all the info in this book. Here is a sample meal plan for three days, for instance:

Day 1
- Breakfast: A serving of Bacon Crusted Frittata Muffins

- Lunch: A serving of Spinach Watercress Keto Salad

- Dinner: A serving of Salmon Patties with Herbs

Day 2

- Breakfast: A serving of Bacon Crusted Frittata Muffins

- Lunch: A serving of Bacon Cheeseburger Salad

- Dinner: A serving of Bacon Cheeseburger Casserole

Day 3

- Breakfast: A serving of Hunger Buster Low Carb Bacon Frittatas

- Lunch: A serving of Spinach Watercress Keto Salad

- Dinner: A serving of Bacon Cheeseburger Casserole

Day 4

- Breakfast: 1 serving of Bacon Crusted Frittata Muffins

- Lunch: 1 serving of Bacon Cheeseburger Salad

- Dinner: 1 serving of Salmon Patties with Herbs

Day 5

- Lunch: 1 serving of Spinach Watercress Keto Salad

- Dinner: 1 serving of Bacon Cheeseburger Casserole

- Breakfast: 2 servings of Hunger Buster Low Carb Bacon Frittatas

Conclusion

The keto diet comes with many benefits. However, what turns many people away is that they will be limited in terms of meal intake. We have provided various forms of keto recipes in this manual. Hence, you can get creative and play around with it.

Besides, the keto lifestyle does not have to be a burden or a restriction. The aim of going into keto diet for many people is to lose weight and enjoy the many health benefits that come along with it. Hence, be sure to follow all you have learned in this book and be creative about how you eat. Diet plan gets boring, and many people find it difficult to stick with it when are restricted to tasteless meals.

Be sure to get your house in order in preparation for the keto lifestyle journey. Get rid of every food that is not keto friendly. If possible, ask your spouse or any of your housemates to join you in the diet. It gets easier if you are not alone. Besides, the absence of keto friendly food also removed the temptation of going above your daily carb limit.

While keto comes with a whole lot of health benefits, users need to be aware of the potential danger. We have listed some class of people not fit for the diet. Besides, if you are on any medication, be sure to talk to your doctor before starting the keto diet. In addition to that, be prepared mentally for the side effects known as keto flu. The good news, however, is that you can lessen the side effect of transition into keto by drinking a lot of water, this is not negotiable.

While the majority of food classes you will concentrate on is fats, be aware that there are good fats and bad fats. Hence, be sure to follow all the recommended ideas in this manual. We have listed bad fats you should stay away from. Keep them in mind, so they do not sabotage your effort to get into ketosis.

On a final note, be aware that you will not likely have the same result with other people, even your spouse if you follow the keto diet together. Keep this in mind, and do not be discouraged. The reason for this is due to the many variables present. Your body, your activity level, and your ages differ. The way you workout and the kind of lifestyle you lead all add to the variables. Be sure to stick to the plan and be faithful with it. When you get to ketosis, you will experience the tremendous health benefits of the keto diet.

References

Calihan J, (2018). Ingredients to avoid on a low-carb or keto diet. Retrieved from https://www.dietdoctor.com/low-carb/ingredients-to-avoid

Eenfeldt, A., (2019). A ketogenic diet for beginners. Retrieved from https://www.dietdoctor.com/low-carb/keto

Freeman J, (2013). Epilepsy's Big Fat Answer. Retrieved from https://www.ncbi.nlm.nih.gov/pmc/articles/PMC3662214/

Fletcher J, (2019). How to get into ketosis fast. Retrieved from https://www.medicalnewstoday.com/articles/324599.php

Hendon L. (2015). Lemon Black Pepper Tuna Salad Recipe [Keto, Paleo, AIP], Retrieved from https://paleoflourish.com/lemon-black-pepper-tuna-salad-keto-paleo-aip/

Joy Filled (No Date). WHITE LASAGNA STUFFED PEPPERS – LOW CARB KETO THM S. Retrieved from https://joyfilledeats.com/white-lasagna-stuffed-peppers/#wprm-recipe-container-13469

Laughing Spatula. (No Date). ZUCCHINI NOODLES WITH SHRIMP. Retrieved from https://laughingspatula.com/zucchini-noodles-with-shrimp/

Lawler M, (2018). Keto and Binge Eating Disorder 101. Retrieved from https://www.everydayhealth.com/ketogenic-diet/keto-binge-eating-disorder/

Levy J, (2018). What Is Ketosis? Hint: It Can Help You Burn Fat & Suppress Your Appetite. Retrieved from https://draxe.com/what-is-ketosis/

Migala J, (2019). A Detailed Guide to the Potential Health Benefits and Risks of the Keto Diet. Retrieved from https://www.everydayhealth.com/diet-nutrition/ketogenic-diet/what-are-benefits-risks-keto-diet/

Moodie A., (no date) Keto Diet for Beginners – Your Complete Guide. Retrieved from https://blog.bulletproof.com/keto-diet-beginners-guide/

Ruled.me, (no date). The Ketogenic Diet - A Keto Guide for Beginners. Retrieved from https://www.ruled.me/guide-keto-diet/

Ruled me. (no date). Ketogenic Diet Food List: Everything You Need to Know. Retrieved from https://www.ruled.me/ketogenic-diet-food-list/

Thrive Strive. (no date)., 7 Benefits of a Keto Diet That You'll Want in Your Life. Retrieved from https://thrivestrive.com/keto-benefits/

Spritzler F. (no date). The complete guide to ketosis. Retrieved from https://www.dietdoctor.com/low-carb/ketosis

William S. (2005). A low-carbohydrate, ketogenic diet to treat type 2 diabetes. Retrieved from https://www.ncbi.nlm.nih.gov/pmc/articles/PMC1325029/

Second Book

Keto Mindset

How to lose weight in 30 days on a Ketogenic diet. Simple steps to Keto success, giving you the best advice and motivation needed from a coach allowing you to achieve long-term results

By Gabriel Walker

Introduction

When I was young, I was that person who ate like an elephant but never picked up weight. That was until I got into my early 20s. As a female, the older you get, the more difficult it is to let go of those few extra pounds. I struggled!

I looked up every diet I could and followed it. I remember trying crazy diets like the Weet-Bix diet and the coffee and no food diet. I even tried water fasting and so many other options, all to no avail. I would stand on the scale and cry every time.

After successfully completing a diet, I quickly ended up picking all that weight right back up again. One day, as I was browsing the Internet, I came across the keto diet. It was something that I didn't really understand at first. It looked like stuff I would love to eat and not the type of food that would send me running for the hills.

After no longer trusting anything I read on the Internet, I was ready to give up and throw in the towel for good. Not long after that my SMS tone went off, and there was a high school reunion coming up that following weekend. I was very anxious to see everyone again. I met up with one of a good friend from high school that very same day, wondering if she would judge the way I looked since I used to be known as the skinny one. When I laid my eyes on her, my jaw dropped! Never in my life would I have thought that my friend whom I haven't seen in a few months was standing right in front of me. She looked amazing! She had lost so much weight, and it was scary!

During our conversation, she informed me about the keto diet and that she was one of the many success stories out there. Then she handed me a handful of sites to visit. I read everything and broke it down for you as much as I could.

I became a keto diet success story myself, and if I can do it, then so can you. But before we even get there, you need to understand why I decided to write this book for you, the readers. I want you to be able to fully understand how your body works and why it is so essential to maintain a healthy lifestyle.

In this book, I am also going to give you my 30-day keto diet plan so that you can start somewhere too. When you do decide to dedicate yourself to this diet, keep in mind it's going to be very hard at first. But I am here to help you along the way. Rome was not built in a day, so be patient with yourself.

I have also included a section on how to increase your metabolism and a few weight loss tips I picked up along the way. If you follow my guide, you are guaranteed to have a long and healthy life with long term results. This is not one of those quick fix me up diets; after a while, it becomes a part of your lifestyle.

Another thing to remember is that when you start any type of diet, it's crucial to also exercise if you haven't already been doing so. Also, if you have a cheat day, don't be too hard on yourself. Generally, people who accidentally or purposely cheat on a diet feel guilty about occasionally having something sweet.

Luckily with this diet, you never have to worry about cheating! Therefore, you will not overeat or do anything you are not supposed to. That is the beauty of this diet. The keto diet is one that will change your life.

I will also suggest some healthy snacks that you can have because I know how difficult it can be in the beginning stages. Eventually, you won't even need these suggestions.

Take my weight loss tips into consideration because I think they are essential to know before you start doing anything. Remember that reliable sites give out recipes too. Once your 30 days are up, you can start moving to other types of keto foods.

Before we even get started, you are probably wondering, "what is a keto diet?" A keto diet is a plan of meals that are very low in carbohydrates. You lower your carbohydrate intake to under 100 grams a day.

This makes it very easy to abolish junk food and all types of heavy processed products. It's important you understand that this is not just a temporary diet; this leads to a lifestyle change.

This is ideal for people with diabetes, people who are overweight or obese, people with many other health reasons, and more! In order for me to prove to you that this diet indeed works, I am going to have to jump into some biology.

Your body's energy

We, as human beings, need the energy to keep us alive. Food breaks down in our bodies and is turned into useable energy. This energy makes us feel awake during the day. The human body has a few places where it gets its energy sources from; some are stored in your body's fats and some in your ketones.

Your body also takes glucose from the liver and all your carbohydrates from the food you eat. Now you may be wondering what will happen if we were to take the carbohydrates away because they are the primary source of energy in your body.

Let me explain this in the simplest way I can.

After you eat your carbs and they enter your bloodstream, they are broken down into glucose. Then, insulin steps in to try and get rid of all the extra glucose from your blood. It takes your glucose and transforms it into glycogen, which is stored primarily in your body's muscles.

This becomes a problem when you don't exercise because the glycogen gets stored in your muscles. When all your muscles are full, and your liver is full, then it sends out a signal to stop the production of insulin.

The glycogen has nowhere to go at this point, so more insulin is released, and eventually, this leads to insulin resistance. When your body reaches this point, the liver sends any left-over glucose to be stored as body fat (Lis, 2019).

This is when you start to gain weight and can develop type 2 diabetes and many other metabolic issues.

Keto snacks

One dill pickle	One slice of bacon	One beef stick	Two stalks of celery
One tablespoon of guacamole	Fifteen pecan nuts	One keto bar	A handful of cherry tomatoes
One hard-boiled egg	One mini round of	Eight brazil nuts	One piece of string cheese

	Babybel cheese		

These are just some of many snacks. These are my go to's because they are my favourites. You can also find different types of snacks; you just have to look them up. Preferably only read the sites that are approved by dieticians. Here are some more snacks that you need to eat in moderation. It all depends on the diet you have.

Below I have compiled a list of grab-to-go snacks. These don't need any preparation, and you can just grab them from your refrigerator when you are hungry.

Olives	Sugar-free jelly
Sugar-free ice cream	Kale chips
Iced coffee	Pork rinds
Sardines	Seaweed snacks
Avocado	Stevia sweetened dark chocolate
Pepperoni slices	Beef jerky
Laughing cow cheese	Macadamia nuts

Below I have compiled a list of the snacks you can make at home. You can find the recipes for them on Google. These do require a bit of preparation, but it is worth it in the long run.

Steak tips	Keto fries
Pizza	Bone broth
Fat bombs	Flaxseed crackers
Keto pate	Keto crisps

Calzones	Salad

Like I mentioned before, these are just some of many snacks. There are many types of snacks, but these are the most popular ones. As you can see, there are many snacks that you fall back on if you get hungry while on this diet.

Remember, a keto diet is a low carbohydrate diet with high-fat content. With this diet, you can reverse type 2 diabetes and treat epilepsy (Lis, 2019), and if that's not why you are here, that's okay too.

This diet is guaranteed weight loss for anyone. The above mentioned are just a bonus!

Chapter 1- Keto diet weight loss tips

Below is a list of weight loss tips, written by Eenfeldt (2019), that are important to follow before, during, and after the diet. These tips helped me better understand a few things when it came to losing weight. I am sure it will do the same for you.

These tips are here to motivate you and encourage you to do the best that you can. Just a friendly warning, you might not see much of a difference in your weight in the first two weeks. This is completely normal. Don't give up, because like I said, these things take time.

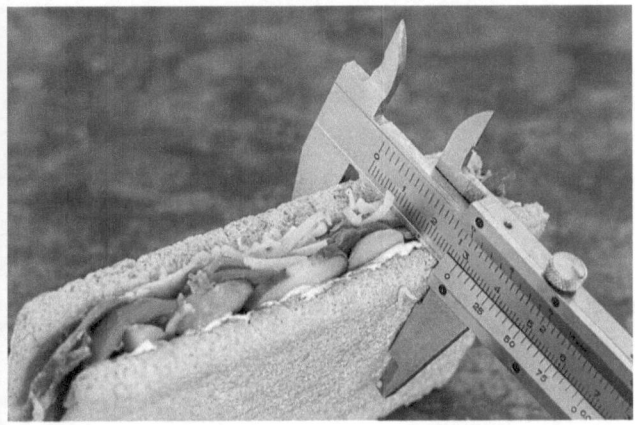

1.   Be persistent

I am going to be super blunt in saying forget about all of those "quick fixes." There is no magic cure to losing weight. It comes with hard work and dedication. You can't simply take a magic pill that will drop those extra pounds overnight. There is absolutely no such thing. It's rubbish and dangerous. So, stay away from those.

Whatever you do, don't starve yourself and think that it is a long-term solution. Starving yourself is dangerous and can lead to bulimia. Don't even attempt to starve yourself just a little bit. This is a horrible way to think you will lose weight successfully.

As soon as you put food in your mouth, your body is going to store that food away because your body does not know when it will get food again. This causes weight gain, and it is simply a bad thing to do to yourself and your body.

You need to understand that your weight did not magically appear on your body overnight. This weight you have on your body has been growing there for many years. It's nothing to be ashamed of, you are reading this for help, and I am going to give it to you. Just be patient with your body; results take time.

Let's get one thing straight, if you want to keep your weight off permanently, you need to change your habits and your lifestyle forever. It's not something you do for a short time and expect it to work. Once you change your lifestyle, everything else will fall into place.

Like I mentioned before, if you don't see a change in the first two weeks, please don't panic. We are all different, and sometimes it takes our bodies longer to adapt to the change. Other people are lucky enough that they start losing weight within the first week.

Work towards losing 1-3kg in the first week. As I said, everyone is different, but work towards that. After that you should be losing half a kilogram a week, all depending on how much excess weight you still have on your body.

You will be happy to know that every kilogram you lose in weight, you lose a centimetre around your bust.

2.   Avoid fruit

Unfortunately, all fruit has sugar that shuts down your fat burning cells in your body. So, it would be best to avoid fruit altogether. When you are eating fruit regularly, it increases your desire to eat, therefore causing your weight loss to slow down rapidly.

If you haven't already guessed it, fruit itself contains a concerning amount of sugar, and we want to stay away from that if we're going to lose weight. Did you know that five servings of fruit contain as much sugar as a 500ml soft drink? That means that sugar is about 50% glucose and 50% fructose.

3.   Eat only when hungry

If you eat when you are hungry, you will be able to limit the need for unnecessary snacking. If you are not hungry during lunchtime, then don't eat lunch. You are more than welcome to skip meals. Try your best not to overeat. This is very easy to do with peanuts.

4.   Review your medicine

The very first thing you need to do when you start your weight loss journey is to check your blood pressure, cholesterol levels, and your sugar to make sure that you are in good health. Many medications can contribute to your struggle of losing weight.

Insulin-releasing tablets	Some contraception medication
Cortisone	Antibiotics
Antipsychotic drugs	Epilepsy drugs
Some anti-depressants	Allergy medication
Insulin injections	Blood pressure drugs

5.   Eat less dairy and nuts

Dairy products slow down weight loss if consumed in large quantities. Nuts, especially salty ones, are very easy to keep eating without realising how much you are consuming. This could be dangerous, as too much salt is not healthy for you either.

6.   Supplement vitamins and minerals

It is nearly impossible to get all the vitamins and minerals we need every single day from just consuming food. Go out and get yourself a high-quality multivitamin that you can take every day. Did you know that it is quite difficult to get vitamin D? The funny thing is that vitamin D is the key to weight loss.

So, look up the right amount of vitamin D that you need to take every single day and buy some in pill form. It should be widely available wherever you are around the world.

7.   Support during your journey

If you are anything like me, you are going to need all the help you can get from friends and family. Have a family meeting and invite your friends over as well.

Tell them what you plan to do and how you are planning to do it.

You never know, your family might decide to join you. The more, the merrier! Once they have all been informed, ask your family and friends for support. Let them know that they are now your pillars. Ask them to encourage you.

8.   Exercise

Your body needs at least one hour of aerobic exercise if you are just starting out. But remember to take it slow and don't overdo it. You still want to be able to walk the next day. If you can, get yourself a smartwatch that tracks the number of steps you take each day.

The average steps for a woman daily is around 10,000 steps. If you are not new to the concept of exercise and you have been consistently doing it, look into joining a dance class or start playing a new sport like tennis.

Remember that exercise is essential every single day!

9.   Check your hormones

If you struggle with losing weight and shedding off those few extra pounds, you should consider getting your thyroid checked. Stress levels, as well as your sex hormones, need to be checked as well. You might not be losing anything due to one of these three problems.

Believe it or not, your hormones play a huge role when it comes to losing weight. If anything is slightly off, it will break your body's equilibrium, and it will not function the way it should. That is why it is imperative to make sure you get these checked as often as possible.

Don't put this off for long; make sure you get regular checkups. Many people don't understand how important these checkups actually are. They could make the world's difference.

10.   Avoid your weekend beer

I personally don't like beer, but many people do. It's better you avoid that weekend beer. That doesn't mean don't drink anything. If you are a man, indulge yourself in some old whiskey. Ladies, stay away from that wine too, have some vodka instead.

Like fruit, beer contains rapidly digested carbs that shut down the fat burning cells in your body. So, you should stay away from the beer altogether. Alcohol, in general, needs to be taken in moderation.

11.   Choose a low carb diet

Studies have shown that when you are on a low carb diet, you burn calories even while you are resting or sleeping. How amazing is that? You can burn up to three hundred calories doing nothing but closing your eyes. You don't even need to move!

Being on a low carb diet means that you need to avoid foods that contain starch and sugar, which includes potatoes, bread, and pasta. The main advantage of a low carb diet is that it makes you full for longer, therefore causing you to eat less. A low carb diet will make you want to eat less in general.

It is also scientifically proven that a low carb diet is the healthiest and most effective way to lose weight. That's why it is best to adopt a low carb diet over any other diet.

12.   Determine if you are really hungry

In today's busy world, even with things changing around us every second, a person can still get bored. Typically, when you are bored and have nothing to do, you start to feel hungry. It's a common feeling for people, especially young adults. You need to make sure that you are not just eating because you have nothing better to do.

Stress is a horrible thing to have. There is absolutely no way to avoid it. There is not a single person on this planet who is not stressed out. You need to see that you are not eating due to stress. Stress eating is like comfort to some people. Try and avoid stress eating at all costs.

Once you have ruled out that you are not doing any of the above, you can then confirm that you are actually hungry and that your body needs food. This tip goes hand in hand with the tip #3. This is helpful to know so that you can decipher if you are really hungry or not.

13.   Stress less

Try yoga or meditation to help ease your restless mind. Meditation doesn't have to take up so much of your time either, 3 to 5 minutes a day to yourself will do you good. Another effective way to de-stress is to pick up a book and read.

Stress releases a horrible hormone called cortisol. This hormone makes you incredibly hungry and causes a substantial change in a person's appetite. This hunger, in the long run, will cause weight gain instead of weight loss.

A respectable amount of relaxation is vital when it comes to staying away from stress. If you feel well rested, you tend to be less stressed out. This, in the long run, will help you avoid stress.

14. Sleep correctly

I am not talking about the way you sleep or the position you sleep in at night. I am talking about the amount of sleep and rest that you get out of it. Remember that you need to get at least fifteen minutes of sunlight a day, not just to get your daily dose of the sun, but it actually contributes to your rest.

If you are a coffee lover, such as myself, I have some bad news for you. Avoid coffee or any sort of caffeine after 1 in the afternoon because caffeine takes forever to leave your system. Also, it would be a great idea to set a bedtime so that you can set a regular routine for yourself.

Rest is vital to losing weight. Once you are in routine, stick to it. This tip goes hand in hand with our previous tip. The point is to avoid stress and get your body relaxed to prevent that stress hormone from being released.

Do not exercise right before you go to bed, as this will keep your body awake, and you will miss out on your beauty sleep. If you have to exercise in the evening, make sure you do so at least four hours before you need to go to sleep.

15. Intermittent fasting

Before we get started with this, I must warn you. Don't do this if you are under the age of 18. Young people should definitely not be doing this as it is not good for their health.

Don't take part in intermittent fasting if you are on any form of medication as this could cause complications for your health. Do not attempt this if you have been diagnosed with chronic stress; this could cause you to faint or pass out.

Lastly, do not attempt this if you suffer from sleep deprivation; this could lead to severe complications. If none of the above applies to you, you can keep reading.

You can keep up with intermittent fasting for as long as you'd like to, so long as you are in good health.

You can do this once a week or every day for a month; the choice is all yours. So, let me break this down for you as much as I can so it's not complicated to understand. The easiest way to do this is to not eat for 16 hours of the day. This includes the hours that you are sleeping. Many people fast from 8pm to 12pm. This means that a person's first meal of the day will be at lunch. You get the idea.

16.   Track your progress

I think that everyone should already know that you should take your measurements before you start on your weight loss journey. After you start your journey, you should only take measurements once a month.

The best time to take your measurements is the very first thing in the morning to get the most accurate results. Your body mass index is the best way to track your weight loss. You don't want to be underweight for your height and age.

The first thing to do is to step on the scale and write down your weight on a piece of paper or in a notebook. After that, grab a measuring tape (the ones they use for sewing) and place it slightly above your belly button. Take a deep breath in and out. Don't try and suck in that tummy of yours! I am watching you!

Make sure the tape fits snug and is not compressing your skin because then you are only cheating yourself. Remember not to feel discouraged; these things take time. Take your measurement in centimetres and write it down.

Remember that for every kilogram you lose, you will lose a centimetre around your bust too!

17.   Weight loss pills

If you have been dieting and it has not been working, only resort to pills as a last resort. Remember, I mentioned that there is no such thing as a magic pill that will make your weight suddenly drop.

It will never make you thin overnight. I'm not saying that these tablets don't work, they do, but only temporarily. Once you stop taking these tablets, all the weight you lost comes back just as quick as you lost it. Most of these weight loss pills are utter rubbish.

The ingredients can cause nasty side effects as well, so take all of this into consideration before deciding to take the first pill you see. You need to do proper and thorough research to make sure what you swallow isn't going to kill you.

18.   Avoid artificial sweeteners

Artificial sweeteners are probably one of the most dangerous products that you can use when it comes to losing weight. They increase a person's appetite immensely and create intense cravings for sweet food. This can also create a bad addiction to sugar, so do your best to steer clear of them.

When I say artificial sweeteners, this includes all and any types of sodas. Diet sodas included, believe it or not. Diet sodas create insulin in your body. This could be very bad for any person; it could lead you to developing type 2 diabetes.

Consumption of artificial sweeteners can be deadly for people with type 1 diabetes. It's best to stay away from any type of sweeteners, artificial or not. It's all dangerous and harmful to your body.

The importance of maintaining a healthy lifestyle

Many people don't consider their lifestyle when they plan to lose weight. In fact, your lifestyle plays a vital role. We as human beings have different views on what a healthy lifestyle is; in our case, it is reaching our optimal physical as well as mental being.

In this day, humans have evolved into leading a lifestyle with very unhealthy habits. Let's be honest with one another, we can live better lifestyles without these habits. These bad habits include smoking cigarettes,drugs, as well as drinking teamed up with very poor and inactive physical activity. This has led us humans to adopt lousy quality diets as well.

To lose weight, you need regular physical activity. So be sure to make yourself a schedule and stick to it. Sleep and rest also play a significant role when it comes to losing those few extra pounds and leading a healthy lifestyle.

Leading a healthy lifestyle is vital for many reasons, including disease prevention. If you do not exercise daily, it leads to sickness and chronic illnesses. Being sick leads you to gain weight due to antibiotics and not getting enough physical exercise.

Leading a healthy lifestyle is important because if you don't watch what you put in your mouth, it can lead you to eat poorly and will cause you to have a chronic poor diet; and if you have a poor diet, you are very likely to pick up various diseases like type 2 diabetes.

If you develop type 2 diabetes, there is a considerable chance that you will gain a lot of weight because insulin releasing medications cause weight gain. You will then also be at risk for heart problems in the near future.

Maintaining a healthy lifestyle is vital to reducing stress and adding on a few more valuable years to your life. This leads me to tell you that if you maintain a healthy lifestyle, you can improve your overall health which includes your mental health.

Important exercises to help you lose weight

Now that we have established that exercising is essential, I would like to share a few weight loss exercises with you. But before I do that, you should know that weight loss exercises are also known as cardiovascular exercises.

The first thing we look at when we want to start training is aerobic exercises. The point of this is to increase your heart rate. This doesn't necessarily mean that you have to run a marathon; it can be walking and swimming too.

Do note that you need to consult your doctor or a personal trainer before attempting exercises on your own. When you are on a low carb diet, you can't dive into extreme exercises without the approval of a professional as it can cause complications.

When you adopt a low carb diet, it puts a lot of stress on your body, so when you do decide to finally exercise, it's important that you listen to your body. You don't want to put yourself in danger just for the sake of losing weight faster.

Please for heaven's sake, make sure you eat enough! Remember, exercising burns carbohydrates first, so you have to be sure that you have enough healthy fats to keep you going.

The first few weeks of your diet are going to be intense, so you should really take it easy by completing low-intensity exercises. This diet works, but I never said it was going to be easy, because if I did, I would be lying to you.

It is challenging to walk past that bakery aisle with all the freshly baked doughnuts and cakes, and it is probably going to drive you insane. But remember why you are doing this. Remember that going on a diet should be for yourself and not anyone else.

Let's take a look at some workouts you can do in a pool. A cardio workout in a pool is pretty simple. When you do decide to go swimming, make sure you follow all the rules when it comes to using a public or gym pool. Swim for five continuous minutes and take a break at the edge of the pool for thirty seconds. Then, grab a kickboard and kick continuously for five minutes. Repeat this exercise three times for a full body and cardio workout (Scott, 2019).

If swimming really isn't your thing, go out and buy a good quality jump rope. Jump for half an hour a day and you are set for a friendly and easy cardio workout. If you have access to a gym, it will probably be best to do some rowing. However, don't overdo it, just row for a little while.

If you have been exercising for a long time and you are comfortable to try more intense training, and you have approval from your doctor or trainer, you can do the following.

If you prefer to exercise at home, I am going to give you my workout plan. You can take two-minute breaks as often as you need to throughout these exercises. The first exercise I usually start with is squats, and I do one hundred and fifty of them. Remember that you can take as many two-minute breaks as you need in between each exercise.

I then proceed to do one hundred lunges, with breaks in-between. Once that is finished, and I have caught my breath, I do one hundred jumping jacks, and eighty leg raises. Once I have caught my breath again, I finish off with some running.

There is an app in the Apple app store that you can download for free. It is called "The Beep Test." The point of the beep test is to reach the finish line before you hear the beep. The speed increases after each beep making the exercise more and more difficult.

Chapter 2- Allowed list of foods for Keto

Now that you have the basics covered, you are probably wondering what exactly it is that you are allowed to eat. Below I am going to share everything I know when it comes to the foods that pass the keto friendly test.

You will be amazed by how many common foods you can eat if you switch around a few of the ingredients. But before I get there, let's start off with the types of meat you are allowed to eat.

You can still have a decent restaurant breakfast anywhere you go because the keto diet is simply that amazing. Take a look below.

Bacon	Cold cuts
Lamb	Fowl
Pork	All red meat
Chicken	Turkey

That might not look like much, but it really is a lot. You will be amazed to know how much fish and seafood you can have as well. I am personally a significant fan of fish, especially squid, so I was happy to learn that I could still eat my favourite seafood. If you are allergic to fish, feel free to skip this section.

All fish	Squid
Scallops	Clams
Oysters	Muscles
Lobster	Shrimp

Crabs	Crawfish

At the beginning of chapter one, I instructed you to avoid fruit at all costs. However, this does not mean that you have to avoid fruit forever. Once you have reached your goal weight, you are more than welcome to start introducing fruit back into your diet; however, do it slowly.

I must admit, I missed avocado for the first few months; but let me tell you, when I got to eat it again, it tasted even better. Consume of these fruits with strict moderation obviously. The keto diet doesn't eliminate everything you love forever, just until you have reached a state of ketosis.

Here is a list of acceptable fruits that you can eat after you have reached your goal.

Raspberries	Strawberry
Lemon	Avocado
Lime	Apricot
Grapefruit	Blackberry

Here is one for all the cheese lovers out there. There is a wide variety of cheeses that you can eat. There are so many options for you to wrap in cold cuts and enjoy! Again, this is all to be taken in moderation. Here are the keto accepted cheeses.

Cheddar	Gouda
Provolone	Mozzarella
Neufchatel	Ricotta
Gruyere	Blue cheese
Parmesan	Fontina
Muenster	Edam

Monterey	Havarti

Next up is a list of salad dressings and fats that you are allowed to have. Most of them have a limit of two tablespoons which still goes incredibly well over a salad of your choice.

Butter	Mayonnaise
Blue cheese dressing	Olive oil
Italian dressing	Avocado oil
Caesar dressing	Coconut oil
Ranch dressing	1000 island dressing

The keto diet even supports those who've adopted a vegan lifestyle. I have compiled a list of vegan protein that you may have if you have decided to live that lifestyle.

Soybeans	Soymilk
Soy nuts	Firm tofu
Tempeh	Silken tofu

There is nothing I love more when it comes to vegetables. You have no idea how ecstatic I was when I found a list of all the veggies I can eat. It is an overwhelming amount, and that made me so happy.

Below I have compiled a list of the many veggies you can have!

Bamboo shoots	Asparagus	Artichoke hearts in water	Artichoke	Romaine lettuce	Radishes
Pumpkin	Okra	Kohlrabi	Daikon	Endive	Radicchio

Onion	Black olives	Leeks	Alfalfa sprouts	Escarole	Bell peppers
Sauerkraut	Spinach	Mushrooms	Broccoli	Arugula	Parsley
Cherry tomato	Tomato	Kale	Brussels sprouts	Bok choy	Jicama
Turnips	Collard greens	Hearts of palm	Cabbage	Celery	Iceberg Lettuce
Green onions	Chard	Eggplant	Cauliflower	Chicory greens	Fennel
Cucumber					

Did you know that with a keto diet you can use all and any spices? If you have cholesterol problems, please don't overuse your salt. It is unhealthy for you.

Moving on, I am going to give you the list that I have compiled for dairy products. This list is a bit short but still worth mentioning.

Unsweetened almond milk	Full fat sour cream	Plain full greek yogurt
Heavy whipping cream	Whole eggs	Egg whites and egg yolk

Now that we have covered all the basics, I am going to add a little extra information in for you to know about. I have also compiled a lovely list of nuts and seeds that you can consume. Unfortunately, the same rule applies as it does to fruit; you should only eat them if you've reached ketosis.

Once you have reached your goal weight, you are more than welcome to start introducing nuts and seeds back into your diet; do so slowly. Here is a list of acceptable nuts and seeds that you can use after you have reached your goal weight.

Peanut butter	Almond butter
Pumpkin seeds	Sunflower seeds
Walnuts	Pistachio nuts
Almonds	Pine nuts
Peanuts	Pecans
Hazelnut	Macadamia nuts

Now that all of our solids have been listed, it's time to move on to liquids. We are going to start off with alcoholic beverages that don't contain carbohydrates. Yes, that's right. Alcohol is keto approved.

Tequila	Gin
Whiskey	Vodka
Rum	Martini

As I mentioned before, beer is a huge no-no; it is like eating loaves of bread one after another. Stick to the list of alcoholic beverages above, and you can still have fun while celebrating special occasions. Next, we have a list of acceptable standard drinks.

Water	Herbal tea
Unsweetened tea	Unsweetened coffee
No calorie flavored seltzers	Sugar-free sparkling water
Diet soda (watch for sweeteners)	Club soda

Now that we have completed the section on foods and drinks that we are allowed to have, the next section is about the foods that we have to stay away from in order to lose weight and reach our goals.

Banned list of foods for Keto

Now, you are probably going to hate what you see here, and sadly the truth hurts, so get ready to have the biggest shock of your life when you finally see everything we are not allowed to eat. Hold on to your seats ladies and gentlemen, this is going to be a rough ride.

Considering we ended on drinks in the previous section, I thought it would be best to start this section off with the drinks we are not allowed to have. This includes alcoholic and non-alcoholic beverages. Here we go.

Wine coolers	Alcopops
Sweetened or flavoured coffee	Sweet cocktails
Sweetened or flavoured tea	Energy drinks
All sweetened drinks	Frozen coffee beverages
Soda	Malt
Juice	Root beer floats
Frappuccino Coffee drinks	Milkshakes

I was so surprised to see that there were so many things that we can't eat when it comes to grains and starches that you normally have with a regular carbohydrate diet. I am going to divide this list into two parts. Let's first have a look at part one.

All whole grains	Any fried food	Whole wheat flour
Oatmeal	French Toast	Rice flour
Cream of wheat	Pasta	Corn flour
Pancakes	Bread	White flour
Waffles	Bagels	Corn starch

Pizza	English muffins	Pasta
Porridge	Croissants	White rice
Barley	Tortilla	Cold breakfast cereals

You will see that the list above contains a lot of baking ingredients and quite a few starches. It is vital that you don't eat any of these as they are not suitable for you and will bring you out of ketosis. Let's now have a look at part two.

Crackers	Muesli
Amaranth	Rye
Millet	Spelt
Quinoa	Bulgur

I put these items in part two because these food items are common misconceptions, in the sense that they are easily mistaken for what some people would call "healthy." They obviously are not. Since we're on the topic of unhealthy foods, I think it's time to move on to the list of fruits you should never eat while on a keto diet.

Dried fruit	Oranges
Kiwifruit	Applesauce
Pears	Dates
Pomegranates	Pears
Pineapple	Plums
Cherries	Figs
Grapes	Banana
Mango	Tangerines

All of these fruits have a high amount of sugar in them, and some even contain starch. It is best to avoid them as much as possible if you want to keep the excess weight off. I have also compiled a list of fruits that contain medium levels of sugar as well as starch-filled fruits.

Apricots	Guava
Honeydew melons	Grapefruit
Apples	Peaches
Nectarines	Papaya
Watermelons	Cantaloupes
Blueberries	

I also compiled a list of vegetables you should not consume. Take a look below.

Lentils	Pinto beans
Lima beans	Baked beans
Black beans	Chickpeas
Kidney beans	Navy beans

If you are not lactose intolerant, you are probably wondering which dairy products we should not consume. You will find that your days for comfort food are over. Here is a hint, no more ice cream!

Ice cream	Yogurt with fruit pieces and sugar
Flavoured dairy	Cottage cheese
Whole and skim milk	Pudding
Soymilk (if you are not a vegan)	Margarine

Now that we are on the topic of comfort foods, there are a few sweets and packaged snacks that we should stay away from. There are also a few processed foods included in there. Remember that all other candy not listed below is also included, as well as all other boxed snacks.

Cupcakes	Twinkies
Cotton candy	Granola bars
Hard candy	Pop-tarts
Chocolate bars	Popcorn
Flavoured nuts	Potato crisps
Pretzels	Tortilla crisps
Rice cakes	Raisins
Breakfast bars	Cheese and cracker snacks

I am going to end this section off with the obvious: you should avoid eating any sugar even if you are not on a diet. This includes all and any types of sugars, honey included, as well as baked goods like cookies and cakes.

Ten common keto mistakes

There are ten common errors that can occur when it comes to losing weight and sticking to a low carb diet.

Overeating protein	Being afraid of fat
Not eating enough	Not exercising
Not eating enough veggies	Being afraid to eat out
Not giving the body enough time to adjust	Listen to friendly advice

Allowing boredom to sabotage your efforts	Not replenishing sodium

Please take the following into consideration. The keto diet allows you to eat eggs; however, that does not mean five or six eggs a day. This will compromise your diet for too much protein. We want to keep with the recommended daily protein.

In order for you to exercise correctly and be healthy, you need to have natural and healthy fats. Don't be afraid of fats; they are good for you. Don't try and get rid of all fats because your body needs them in order for it to function normally.

People think that when they are on this diet plan that they are not meant to eat a lot of food. That is a common mistake made by many people. You have to eat as much as is necessary so that you don't pass out or cause severe damage to your body. It is crucial that you eat!

Remember that lovely long list of veggies I gave you earlier? You know you don't have to eat them raw, right? Use spices and melt the right amount of recommended cheese over top of them! This is allowed. Just make sure you eat an appropriate serving of veggies.

Like I said before, Rome was not built in a day. You have to give your body time to adjust. It is a life-altering diet and to make sure you get the results you want, you're going to have to be patient and give your body all the time it needs to adjust.

This also means that you have to be mindful throughout this process; you are working hard to make a lifestyle change, so don't let your efforts be destroyed by boredom or stress. I used to eat a lot when I was stressed, and unfortunately, my to that was biggest downfall. Don't allow this happen to you too!

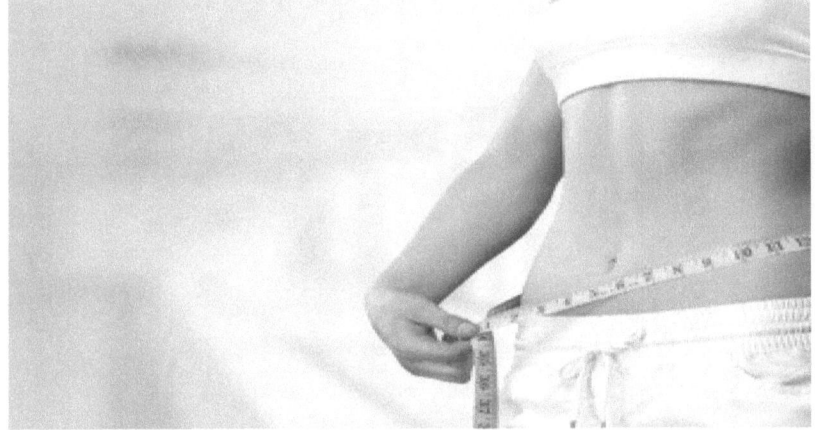

Many people are going to want to give you advice; it is even better if this comes from people who have successfully completed this type of diet. But that doesn't mean that you shouldn't listen to friendly advice from other people. Any useful information is considered advice, use it or don't; it is entirely up to you.

Chapter 3- 30-day meal plan

This chapter is all about the meal plans I have drawn up. This is a 30-day keto diet plan and has been proven successful for weight loss.

There are so many recipes that can fall into this meal plan, so don't be shy to do some research on how to make them. You will see that pizza and other greasy-like foods are still listed on this meal plan. This is because you can still make them with different ingredients from what the original recipe uses.

Day	Breakfast	Lunch	Dinner
Monday	Bacon spinach casserole	Spicy beef salad	Prawns zucchini linguini
Tuesday	Egg salad	Green beans pork stir fry	Burger pancakes
Wednesday	Oopsie bread breakfast sandwich	Smoked chicken salad	Pork bombs with brie
Thursday	Bacon egg cups	Chicken bacon crustless quiche	Smoked haddock casserole
Friday	Ham cheese rolls	Taco mince with crispy cheese	Meatballs in creamy tomato sauce
Saturday	Mini egg muffins	Cauliflower chicken cheesy skillet	Meatloaf

Day	Breakfast	Lunch	Dinner
Sunday	Smoked pancetta crustless quiche	Tuna salad	Stuffed chicken rolls
Day	**Breakfast**	**Lunch**	**Dinner**
Monday	Chia pudding	Shrimp and cauliflower salad	Low carb burgers
Tuesday	Devilled eggs	Spaghetti squash	Low carb pizza
Wednesday	Classic bacon and eggs	Chicken and mashed cauliflower	Salmon with pesto sauce
Thursday	Cauliflower hash browns	Portabella burgers	Steak and garlic kale
Friday	Omelettes	Low carb spaghetti	Eggplant pizza
Saturday	Lox and cream cheese on flax crackers	Garlic shrimp and spinach salad	Low carb lasagna
Sunday	Pancakes low carb style	Steak and mushroom lettuce wraps	Mozzarella meatballs
Day	**Breakfast**	**Lunch**	**Dinner**
Monday	Waffles low carb style	Turkey lettuce wraps	Shakshuka
Tuesday	Smoked salmon with cream cheese, tomato, and	Roast beef salad	Pizza frittata

Day	Breakfast	Lunch	Dinner
	onion		
Wednesday	Green smoothie	Bacon chef's salad	Tuna casserole
Thursday	Egg with salsa and cheese	Low carb chilli with beef	Steak and potato salad
Friday	Egg bake and skillets with meat and veggies	Bacon crunch brussels sprouts	Zucchini shrimp scampi
Saturday	Peanut butter on flax crackers	Chicken and zucchini poppers	Low carb lettuce wrap tacos
Sunday	Guacamole and bacon with eggs	Low carb french fries	Low carb stuffed peppers

Day	Breakfast	Lunch	Dinner
Monday	Lox and cream cheese on flax crackers	Zucchini patties	Strawberry spinach chicken salad
Tuesday	Tuna salad on cucumbers	Baked salmon with lemon garlic butter	Pork roast with crispy asparagus
Wednesday	Coconut porridge	Bacon mushroom cheeseburger lettuce wraps	Chicken breast with herb butter
Thursday	Oopsie bread breakfast sandwich	Stuffed tomatoes	Mozzarella mushroom and chicken bake
Friday	Bacon egg	Low carb meat	Sushi feast

	cups	pie	
Saturday	Ham cheese rolls	Steak with bearnaise sauce	Lamb roast with herbs and cream cheese
Sunday	Mini egg muffins	Grilled polish sausage with cabbage	Low carb chicken quesadillas

Remember, at the beginning of chapter one, I mentioned that you might not see much of a difference in the first two weeks. This is completely normal. Don't give up, because like I said, these things take time. Try your best and don't get discouraged.

These foods don't taste bad at all, and they are worth your time to prepare. You will begin to have a lot more energy and you will wake up in a better mood than you usually would. In order for you to mentally and physically accept this lifestyle, you need to think of this as a treat to your body.

It doesn't help if you feel like you are being punished. A negative mindset and pessimistic thoughts are not going to help you at all. You need to do your best to remain positive. Remember you are doing this for yourself.

Chapter 4- The science behind the keto weight loss

At the beginning of this book, I mentioned that we need energy to keep us alive. The reason we eat food is so that our bodies can break it down and turn it into useable energy, which will in turn keep us energized throughout the day.

The human body is an amazing thing. A lot of its energy is stored in the body's fats and ketones. Your body also retrieves the glucose from the liver and all your carbohydrates from the food you eat.

Now you might recall what happens when we take away carbohydrates; that's right, your body will reach a state of ketosis.

After you eat any food containing carbohydrates, and it has entered your bloodstream, it is readily broken down into what we call glucose. Then, your body's insulin steps in to try and remove all the excess glucose from your bloodstream. It then takes your glucose and turns it into glycogen, which is stored primarily in your body's muscles.

All the stored glycogen then can cause problems if you don't exercise regularly. It runs out of space in the muscles and uses the last space in the liver, your liver will then send out a signal to stop the production of insulin.

It is at this point that the glycogen has nowhere to go, so more and more insulin is distributed into your bloodstream, and this without a doubt leads to insulin resistance. When your body is at this point, the liver transfers any left-over glucose to be stored as body fat.

This is when you start to gain weight and develop type 2 diabetes as well as many other metabolic issues.

This is the beauty of this diet; this diet reprograms your body and can even help with common illnesses such as polycystic ovarian syndrome and irritable bowel syndrome.

Typically ketones have no role in giving the body energy or producing it either. For those of you who don't know what ketones and ketone bodies are, I am going to provide you with a definition by Wikipedia, along with a simple interpretation as it can get a little confusing ("Ketone bodies," n.d.).

"Ketone bodies have three molecules (acetoacetate, beta-hydroxybutyrate and the spontaneous breakdown product of acetoacetate, acetone) containing the ketone group that is formed by the liver by fatty acids during periods of low food intake, restrictive carbohydrate diets, starvation, lengthy forceful exercise, boozing or in untreated type 1 diabetes."

To sum that up in simple terms, ketones are produced by the liver during a normal carbohydrate diet, which is similar to fasting for long periods of time.

"Ketone bodies are willingly transported into tissues outside the liver and converted into acetyl-CoA, which then enters the citric acid cycle and is oxidised in the mitochondria for energy. In the brain, ketone bodies are also used to make acetyl-CoA into long-chain fatty acids."

Ketone bodies are transported into tissues and then converted into a long chain of fatty acids.

"Ketone bodies are formed by the liver under the circumstances listed above as a product of powerful gluconeogenesis, which is the production of glucose from non-carbohydrate sources."

"They are thus continuously unrestricted into the blood by the liver together with newly formed glucose after the liver glycogen stores have been exhausted; this happens within the first 24 hours."

"When two acetyl-CoA molecules lose their A groups they can form a (covalent) dinner called acetoacetate. Beta-hydroxybutyrate remains a compact system of acetoacetate, in which the ketone group is transformed into an alcohol group."

"Both are four carbon molecules, that can eagerly be changed back into acetyl-CoA by utmost tissues of the body, with the distinguished allowance of the liver. Acetone is the decarboxylated form of acetoacetate which cannot be converted back into acetyl-CoA except via detoxification in the liver where it is converted into lactic acid, which can, in turn, be oxidised into pyruvic acid, and only then into acetyl-CoA."

"Ketone bodies have a distinctive smell, which can easily be spotted in the smell of persons in ketosis and ketoacidosis. It is often labelled as fruity or like nail polish remover (which usually contains acetone or ethyl acetate)."

"Apart from the three endogenous ketone bodies, acetone, acetoacetic acid, and beta-hydroxybutyric acid, other ketone bodies like beta-keto pentanoate and beta-hydroxypentanoate possibly will be formed as a result of the metabolism of synthetic triglycerides, such as triheptanoin."

Ketone and ketone bodies are not the same thing. ketones, as defined by Wikipedia, are:

"In chemistry, a ketone is an animate compound with the structure $RC(=O)R'$, where R and R' can be an assortment of carbon-containing substituents. Ketones and aldehydes are pure compounds that contain a carbonyl group (a carbon-oxygen double bond).

They are considered 'simple' because they do not have reactive groups like –OH or –Cl attached directly to the carbon atom in the carbonyl group, as in carboxylic acids containing –COOH. Many ketones are acknowledged, and many are of high position in the industry and in biology. Examples include many sugars (ketoses) and the manufacturing solvent acetone, which is the smallest ketone" ("Ketones," n.d.).

Lipolysis and Ketosis

Under normal circumstances, ketones have no business giving the body energy. But when you are on the keto diet, ketones are in charge of energy levels, and at the same time, start the automatic fat burning switch.

When carbs vanish, the body goes into a state called lipolysis, which is scientifically proven to be in direct correlation with weight loss. The body is forced to use the fat stored in your muscles and melts it off the body, which is referred to as ketosis.

Ketosis and keto acids are two different concepts. Ketosis is a natural fat burning process while keto acids is what arises in diabetes; that is why keto acids are very dangerous (Lis, 2019).

Benefits of the Ketogenic Diet

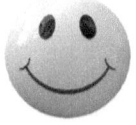

There is an overwhelming amount of advantages you can

get from this diet and lifestyle. The first advantage is weight loss. It has been proven in a number of studies that eating low carbs results in weight loss. This has been verified by the thousands of people, like me, who have struggled with weight.

Keto diet eliminates cravings you have on a day to day basis. It stabilizes your blood sugar levels and your appetite. It also lowers your levels of visceral fat, which is your belly fat and the excess fat surrounding your organs. As a result, your blood pressure will also be lowered, which will make it less likely that you experience a stroke or heart attack.

Keto diet also has the benefit of reducing the risk of heart disease, diabetes, and cancer. This diet is also used to treat several types of cancer and slows down the growth of tumours in the body. It is also used to treat brain injury, Parkinson's disease, epilepsy, Alzheimer's disease, and Polycystic ovarian syndrome (Lis, 2019).

The ketogenic diet increases your protein intake, which has a lot of benefits for your body. It also limits your carbohydrate consumption, which means you have a smaller variety of foods to choose from to eat, resulting in weight loss.

Chapter 5- Increasing your metabolism on the keto diet

When you start the keto diet, you might feel like your metabolism has taken a step back. There is nothing to worry about because this section is here for if you need it. There are also strips you can buy to test your level of ketosis, which will help you determine what your metabolism is like at its current stage.

Once you see that you are in the ketosis phase, this means that your metabolism is at its best it can be. If the results are opposite of that, that is when you look for ways to kick start your metabolism in order to reach ketosis. Below are seven tips you can follow to try and reach your desired level of ketosis (Fletcher, 2019).

Let's take a look at these and remember, if you keep eating correctly, there will not be a need to do this. If you are struggling, then I am here to help you.

1. Increase your physical activity

This one is first on the list because it's most important. In the beginning, I told you to take it easy unless you get the go-ahead from your doctor or personal trainer. If you haven't reached somewhere close to ketosis within the first month and a half, there is a possibility that you are not exercising enough.

2. Reducing carbohydrate intake

If you decided to start the diet off with just 20 grams of carbs a day, you might want to cut that down to about half. It is possible that your body is still consuming too many carbohydrates and that will, without a doubt, cause a problem with your metabolism. So, reduce your carb intake.

3. Fasting for short periods

If you haven't decided to fast yet, now might be a good time to do this. Start off fasting one day a week and see what that does for you. If you see no changes, increase it two days a week but don't fast one day after the other; this can be dangerous. Fast for short periods of time. I'm sure that if you do this, you will be able to see the results.

4. Increase your healthy fats

It's important you include foods in your diet that are considered healthy fats. An example of healthy fats are an avocado and nuts. You can also cook food using flaxseed oil, coconut oil, or a basic virgin olive oil.

5. Test your ketone levels

You can have your ketones tested through a blood test. A blood test may not be your only option, but it is by far the easiest. A blood test will give you all the information you need. Get a blood test form from your general practitioner and visit your nearest blood clinic; it's that easy!

6. Maintain a high protein intake

Remember what I mentioned earlier about watching your protein intake and levels. If you are still struggling with this, it's likely that you are not getting enough protein to sustain ketosis. You will lose muscle mass instead of gaining, and that should be your first warning sign.

7. Use coconut oil

This is an excellent investment. The easiest way to reach ketosis is through the use of coconut oil. This one goes hand in hand with tip #4. If you do both correctly, you won't have a problem reaching your weight goals. Coconut oil isn't very hard to find, and it's generally inexpensive. It's very good for you, and it will make your life a hell of a lot easier.

Generally, if you have reached ketosis, you already know that you simply have to follow the same routine every day. However, we are all human and we sometimes make mistakes, and that's totally okay.

Remaining positive throughout your journey

There will be days where you will feel like none of this is worth it and that you are wasting your time. However, I can promise you that it will all be worth it in the end.

Male or female, come hell or high water I have faith in you, and I believe you can do this! If you are really struggling with motivation, set yourself a goal board. Take an A5 piece of cardboard and stick your goals on there, so that every time you feel like giving up, you will be reminded of what you are working towards.

I can proudly say I lost over 20 kilograms after adopting this lifestyle, and I have never felt better. I don't feel like I lack energy, and I am actually excited to wake up in the mornings because I feel good about myself.

This lifestyle has wholly built up my self-image, and I have finally escaped the depression that had been weighing me down for 19 years. Your mental health is just as important as your physical health, so it's important you take charge of your life now.

Many people these days suffer from low self-esteem, and I can guarantee that at one point in your life, you have felt terrible about yourself. But once you start losing all that extra weight, you start to feel really good about yourself.

Clothes that used to be too small will now fit comfortably, and you will be able to live a long and healthy life the same way that I am. It makes the world's difference, so go and grab some paper and cut out pictures for inspiration and motivation or write down your goals.

Every time you want to give up and throw in the towel, just know that this is a normal reaction, but once you get past that, you will see that the results will change your life forever.

10 things you need to know about the keto diet

As with any diet, there are things you need to know beforehand. Things that you might find strange but that are completely normal. The following list will provide you with 10 additional facts about the keto diet ("The Top 10 Things," 2019):

1. Keto can treat medical conditions

As you might recall, a keto diet can in fact treat grave medical conditions.

2. Eating keto foods doesn't have to be expensive

Some diets can become very expensive; however, a keto diet doesn't have to be. Now that you have a list of what you can and can not eat, you can go and buy your ingredients in bulk, thereby saving money.

3. Keto is more than just a diet

This is true on so many levels. It helps manage diseases such as those listed earlier in the book. It's not just a diet, and it's also not something you can start then stop; it becomes a part of your lifestyle.

4. Keto customization

You can adjust your keto diet to the way your body works and how your body processes carbohydrates. You need to figure out what works for you and stick to it.

5. Keto takes time

As I have mentioned so many times already, it might take a few days before you notice any changes. All the stories you hear of people dropping weight like it's hot is simply because they had more excess weight to lose than you do. So, be patient.

6. Ketosis is different for everyone

Unfortunately, no human being's body works in the same way; so no two people will lose the same amount of weight at the same time. This is physically impossible.

7. Keto flu is a real thing

You think you might be picking up the flu, right? Wrong! This is your body's way of adjusting to the change. You might feel sore and feel like you have the flu, but you really do not.

8. Keto breath is real

The scent of your breath will change as it adapts to your new lifestyle. Some have described the smell to be similar to acetone (nail polish remover). Remember to brush those pearly whites and carry around breath mints; it's a small price to pay!

9. Keto will affect your workouts

Like I said previously, in the beginning stages of the diet, complete your workouts at a low intensity. If you were a daily exerciser prior to the keto diet,, the speed at which you complete exercises will change and you may become slower. However, it will get a lot easier as you progress further into your diet. So, don't worry, you'll get to the intensity you were once at really soon.

10.   Keto farts

This diet can cause a build-up of a lot of gas. Depending on who you are and what you eat, the intensity will vary. Your stomach will be adjusting, so don't be surprised by the gas.

Conclusion

Now that we have reached the end of our journey together, I would like to take this opportunity to thank you for taking the time for me to give you all the valuable information that you need on your keto journey.

Let's review everything that we have covered, right from the very start.

- Keto diet and weight loss tips

1. Be persistent

2. Avoid fruit

3. Eat only when hungry

4. Review your medicine

5. Eat less dairy and nuts

6. Supplement vitamins and minerals

7. Support during your journey

8. Exercise

9. Check your hormones

10. Avoid your weekend beer

11. Choose a low carb diet

12. Determine if you are really hungry

13. Stress less

14. Sleep correctly

15. Intermittent fasting

16. Track your progress

17. Weight loss pills

18. Avoid artificial sweeteners

- The importance of maintaining a healthy lifestyle

- Important exercises to help you lose weight

- Allowed foods for keto

- Banned foods for keto

- Ten common keto mistakes

- 30-day meal plan

- The science behind keto weight loss

- Lipolysis and Ketosis

- Benefits of the Keto diet

- Increasing your metabolism on the keto diet

1. Increasing your physical activity

2. Reducing carbohydrate intake

3. Fasting for short periods

4. Increase your healthy fats

5. Test your ketone levels

6. Maintain high protein intake

7. Use coconut oil

- Remaining positive throughout your journey

- 10 things you need to know about the keto diet

As you can see, we have come a very long way together. If this process is followed, the success rate is 100%. All you need is motivation and a love for the lifestyle.

With all of this information, you are guaranteed to lose weight and become another success story. Remember to be patient with yourself.

If you are one of the lucky ones, you will lose most of your excess weight within the first week. Remember to take it easy with your exercises and don't be afraid to eat your food.

Remember to check in with a professional to make sure that this diet is suitable for you depending on your current health.

The keto lifestyle isn't for everyone. But if you push through, you will receive all the benefits and more.

Don't give up on yourself, remember your goal board, and don't get discouraged when results don't appear as quickly as you'd like them to.

Remember that once your 30 days are up, you can go and look for other keto-friendly recipes so you can enjoy your food, your life, and the brand new you!

If you liked this guide leave me a comment on Amazon!

Thank you!!!

Citations

Ayuda, T. (2019). *10 Calorie-Torching Exercises to Do If You Want to Lose Weight.* [online] Prevention. Available at: https://www.prevention.com/weight-loss/a20474562/best-weight-loss-exercises/ [Accessed 20 May 2019].

Dr. Andreas Eenfeldt, M. (2019). *How to Lose Weight – The Top 18 Simple Tips – Diet Doctor.* [online] Diet Doctor. Available at: https://www.dietdoctor.com/how-to-lose-weight#2 [Accessed 20 May 2019].

Dr. Anthony Gustin, M. (2019). *47 Healthy Keto Snacks That Won't Kick You Out of Ketosis.* [online] Perfect Keto. Available at: https://perfectketo.com/ultimate-healthy-keto-snack-list/ [Accessed 20 May 2019].

Pixabay.com. (2019). *Free Image on Pixabay - Acetone, Ketone, Carbonyl Group.* [online] Available at: https://pixabay.com/illustrations/acetone-ketone-carbonyl-group-2876278/ [Accessed 20 May 2019].

Pixabay.com. (2019). *Free Image on Pixabay - Food, Diet, Keto, Ketodieta.* [online] Available at: https://pixabay.com/photos/food-diet-keto-ketodieta-fitness-3223286/ [Accessed 20 May 2019].

Pixabay.com. (2019). *Free Image on Pixabay - Salad, Fresh, Food, Diet, Health.* [online] Available at: https://pixabay.com/photos/salad-fresh-food-diet-health-374173/ [Accessed 20 May 2019].

Pixabay.com. (2019). *Free Image on Pixabay - Smiley, Emoticon, Dash Face, Grin.* [online] Available at: https://pixabay.com/illustrations/smiley-emoticon-dash-face-grin-1020193/ [Accessed 20 May 2019].

Pixabay.com. (2019). *Free Image on Pixabay - Yoga, Meditation, Spiritual, Mental.* [online] Available at: https://pixabay.com/vectors/yoga-meditation-spiritual-mental-153436/ [Accessed 20 May 2019].

Frey, M. (2019). *The 3 Types of Exercise You Need to Lose Weight.* [online] Verywell Fit. Available at: https://www.verywellfit.com/types-of-exercise-for-weight-loss-3495992 [Accessed 20 May 2019].

Katherine Marengo LDN, R. (2019). *7 fast and effective ways to get into ketosis.* [online] Medical News Today. Available at:

https://www.medicalnewstoday.com/articles/324599.php [Accessed 20 May 2019].

En.wikipedia.org. (2019). *Ketone*. [online] Available at: https://en.wikipedia.org/wiki/Ketone [Accessed 20 May 2019].

En.wikipedia.org. (2019). *Ketone bodies*. [online] Available at: https://en.wikipedia.org/wiki/Ketone_bodies [Accessed 20 May 2019].

Lis, N. (2019, January 03). Keto Diet Guide for Beginners. Retrieved from https://lowcarbbabe.com/keto-diet-guide-beginners-download/

Morgan, H. (2019). *Importance of Living a Healthy Lifestyle | Livestrong.com*. [online] LIVESTRONG.COM. Available at: https://www.livestrong.com/article/31783-importance-lifestyle/ [Accessed 20 May 2019].

Scott, J. (2019). *Getting a Workout in the Pool Can Be Easy for Beginners*. [online] Verywell Fit. Available at: https://www.verywellfit.com/swimming-for-beginners-weight-loss-advice-3496001 [Accessed 20 May 2019].

KetoLogic. (2019). *The Top 10 Things You Need to Know Before Going Keto - KetoLogic*. [online] Available at: https://ketologic.com/article/the-top-10-things-you-need-to-know-before-going-keto/ [Accessed 20 May 2019].